# DON'T LET THEM HIDE THEIR
# SMILE

The Guide to Orthodontic Care for Your Child

# DON'T LET THEM HIDE THEIR
# SMILE

## MICHAEL J. WILSON, DDS

Published by Advantage, Charleston, South Carolina.
Member of Advantage Media Group.

ADVANTAGE is a registered trademark, and the Advantage colophon is a trademark of Advantage Media Group, Inc.

Printed in the United States of America.

10 9 8 7 6 5 4 3 2 1

ISBN: 978-1-64225-006-0
LCCN: 2017964414

Cover design by George Stevens.
Layout design by Megan Elger.

This publication is designed to provide accurate and authoritative information in regard to the subject matter covered. It is sold with the understanding that the publisher is not engaged in rendering legal, accounting, or other professional services. If legal advice or other expert assistance is required, the services of a competent professional person should be sought.

 Advantage Media Group is proud to be a part of the Tree Neutral® program. Tree Neutral offsets the number of trees consumed in the production and printing of this book by taking proactive steps such as planting trees in direct proportion to the number of trees used to print books. To learn more about Tree Neutral, please visit **www.treeneutral.com**.

Advantage Media Group is a publisher of business, self-improvement, and professional development books. We help entrepreneurs, business leaders, and professionals share their Stories, Passion, and Knowledge to help others Learn & Grow. Do you have a manuscript or book idea that you would like us to consider for publishing? Please visit **advantagefamily.com** or call **1.866.775.1696**.

# TABLE OF CONTENTS

# Foreword

# From the Founder of Excellence in Orthodontics

My name is Dr. Dustin Burleson. I'm an orthodontist and the founder of Excellence in Orthodontics. My reasons for becoming an orthodontist and forming a national organization for exceptionally successful orthodontists leading the field in both clinical and patient care—instead of becoming a veterinarian or handsome movie actor or professor of poetry—are easily found at ExcellenceinOrthodontics.org, if you're curious. They might matter to you.

But this book is about *you*, the parent, and your son or daughter, not about me. It's about information you need to know to make intelligent, responsible decisions about your child's health, appearance, self-esteem, and social interactions ... of a permanent, lifelong nature. Does your child really *need* braces? If so, when? If so, who should you trust to provide his orthodontic care? How will you know you're not being ripped off?

This book isn't *Fifty Shades of Gray*. It just can't be that exciting. But if you take the time to read this book, you'll know how to confidently and correctly make whatever decisions you need to make about your child's orthodontic care.

It's *not* 1982.

To start, we're no longer dealing with heavy, ugly, tight, painful metal braces—every visit to have them tightened was another round of torture; they were hard to put on, hard to keep on, painful to remove, and it was irritating having a list of foods and activities to avoid for a long period of time. If your child needs braces now, the experience won't be anything like it was when you were a kid. He won't even try hiding under the bed and have to be dragged kicking and screaming to the car to visit my office.

Not only has *everything* about braces changed, but now all braces are created differently. So try to get that horrible, metal-mouth image out of your head. You're probably aware of invisible braces, maybe by a brand name: Invisalign. That's what prompts a lot of patients to call or email me in the first place. However, Invisalign is but one of a number of options to be considered to get to *the* best, customized, and personalized answer to your child's needs. You don't want to equate this to buying something over the counter: "Hey, give me Invisalign. How much?" It's more complicated than that. But it's a good representation of modern braces. They can be (nearly) invisible, pliable and with lighter steel, safer, and even self-removable for hygiene or sports and easily put back in place. They're not painful and achieve more certain results in a shorter period of time.

When I was growing up, a lot of kids didn't get braces they really needed and their parents let them off the hook, either because they believed their child couldn't tolerate the pain or because the cost was just beyond the family's budget. Now that braces are virtually painless, what about the cost?

Today's far better braces cost *less* than the one-size-fit-all, metal-mouth braces of the '60s, '70s, and '80s. They cost as little as one Starbucks drink a day for a year, rarely more than twice that, and there are a number of different payment plans available if needed. So, that second hurdle is a lot lower than it was when our parents encountered it.

In other words, the first of my two introductory messages is: *relax.*

I've got your back. It's going to be okay—better than okay, easier than okay, and more convenient than okay. Orthodontic procedures *won't* hurt your child, and he or she will surprise you by not complaining it does. It's *not* going to hurt your bank account; you won't be reduced to a backyard stay-cation next summer and the summer after that. It's *not* going to be a maddening maelstrom of appointments of uncertain length, or hours in a waiting room. Not at *my* office.

## More Than Just Braces

My second introductory message is: this is about more than just braces.

Orthodontic care for a child, preteen, or teen is more than just correcting crooked, crowded teeth with braces. That's like thinking diabetes only needs attention when feet have to be amputated, or getting tires checked might be a good idea after being stranded with a flat at night while it's pouring rain.

*"We really appreciated the care and attention we received, and the explanations of the processes that you undertook to correct Daniels underbite. The payment plans were really exceptional and affordable!"*

**—SHELBY D.**

Orthodontic checkups *by an orthodontist*[1], starting at age seven are a proper part of child rearing. In many cases, prevention is less troublesome and less costly. Even if you're late getting your son or daughter in, it's still possible they won't need braces and that other treatment options will do. But if they do need braces, the sooner you know of the options, the better.

This is also about more than just braces because it impacts psychological and emotional health, not just oral health. This is discussed later in the book.

## Why It's Important

1.  Straight teeth function better, are easier to clean, and are more likely to last a lifetime.

2.  People with straight, well-aligned teeth can avoid gum disease, which has very serious health ramifications.

3.  Properly aligned jaws reduce the risk of temporomandibular joint disorders (TMJ), which can ruin sleep or cause chronic headaches or migraines.

4.  Both kids and adults with great smiles feel better about themselves, and that can greatly increase their confidence.

Some parents put off orthodontic treatment, but these irregularities and problems do *not* heal themselves. *This isn't acne; they don't grow out of it.* The problems only grow worse and harder to resolve with age.

---

1   All orthodontists are dentists, but dentists are *not* the same as or suitable substitutes for orthodontists. Read on to find out more.

# Don't Let Them Hide Their Smile

Never smiling isn't easy in an age of selfies and social media. Children can become self-conscious—painfully self-conscious—and embarrassed. "No thanks, Mom, I'd rather just stay home."

Teen suicide has skyrocketed since social media shaming and bullying rose to ugly prominence. Teen depression affects everything from getting the good grades needed to get into a good college to first dates, first loves, and enjoying (or hating) their childhood and teen years. But it doesn't stop there. Uncorrected, bad smiles go with them to college and into their career.

This isn't just cosmetic either. It's also medical and can be a serious detriment to their health.

So, read on. Be informed. Be able to ask smart questions and do the right thing. I guarantee you'll be much better able to correctly and confidently make good choices for your family through this book.

**Dr. Dustin S. Burleson, DDS**

*Founder, Excellence in Orthodontics*

*Clinical Professor, The University of Missouri Kansas City School of Dentistry, Department of Graduate Orthodontics & Dentofacial Orthopedics*

*Adjunct Professor, The Children's Mercy Hospital, Kansas City, Missouri, Department of Cleft & Craniofacial Orthodontics*

*Director, The Rheam Foundation for Cleft & Craniofacial Orthodontics*

# Introduction

Many of my patients ask me the question, "What made you become an orthodontist?" My inspiration came from my own experiences as a kid with "buck" teeth. I didn't mind them so much—I'd mastered the art of squirting water through the gaps in them at my brother, which was a win as far as I was concerned—but thankfully my parents decided to put me in braces when I was about fourteen.

I didn't really know what to expect from my new orthodontist, Dr. Wright, but he and his staff made office visits a fun experience. They were so welcoming and friendly. He always remembered my name, what grade I was in, and what my interests were. He cared about me as a person, not just a set of teeth he was straightening. They always sent me a card on my birthday, which amazed me, and I remember that they also made it easy for my parents to afford treatment, which made them happy. When my braces came off, my smile looked a lot better and I felt more confident. I remember thinking, "This is a cool way to make a living."

That experience propelled me into ten years of school at the University of Buffalo, New York, where I completed the four years of school for my undergraduate degree, an additional four years for my dental degree, and a final two years for my orthodontic residency. During my residency, I visited my parents who had moved to North Carolina and decided pretty quickly that I liked their winters better than the ones in Buffalo. So, after graduating, I moved to North Carolina and went into practice with two older orthodontists, ultimately starting my own practice in 2004 in Durham, North Carolina, with a second location in Oxford, North Carolina.

Dr. Wright's great example is one I've tried to emulate. About 70 percent of the patients we see are adolescents and younger, and my team and I make sure that each one of them feels as special and appreciated as Dr. Wright made me feel.

Ideally, I like to see children initially when they're about seven. While we don't treat them at that age outside of some special cases, it's important to establish a baseline early on so we can assess where they are and help their parents understand what potential issues they may have down the line. Our Kids' Club is a way to make that observation program fun, as we monitor their growth and development until the appropriate time for treatment. We'll see our Kids' Club members about every six to nine months, take images as needed, and update our notes, all at no charge. This helps kids get familiar with the office and comfortable with me, and also gives their parents time to plan for the process financially. Kids even get their own rewards cards, where they can earn points for losing baby teeth or doing well on their report cards. Our focus on children may be why we regularly get whole families coming through our practice—and very often,

Mom and Dad too, once their children have finished their treatment. We also offer family discounts to make it more affordable.

The best thing about my job is getting to know these families, and seeing the positive impact my work has on their lives. One young lady we're treating now started with us when she was ten. She was very shy when she first met us, and would barely open her mouth to speak. She used to need her mom or dad to be with her when she was in the chair, to hold her hand and talk for her. Now, she's almost ready to get her braces off, and she leaves her parents in the waiting room. She talks and engages my team members; she even laughs and smiles during her appointment—and for her, that's tremendous progress that reminds us of the amazing profession we are part of.

As people learn about all the new technology making orthodontics easier and faster, we're seeing more adults come in for consultations who want their teeth straightened. Invisalign is particularly attractive to them, since many of them are a little self-conscious about being seen in braces, and they like the many advantages Invisalign offers in terms of comfort and easy care. My oldest patient is seventy-six; in her case, her decision to get her teeth straightened had to do with an accident that had knocked her bite out of whack, but most of my older patients are there because they've finally decided to get the smiles they'd always wanted. Even a retired dentist came to me to get his teeth straightened!

And of course, our work isn't just about appearances; teeth that don't fit together properly may abnormally wear down, and are often harder to properly clean, so your teeth won't last the way they should. People often put off dealing with bad bites or other orthodontic issues because they're afraid of the cost of treatment. So often when they come to see us, they're pleasantly surprised at how affordable braces are, and how much shorter treatment times are nowadays than they used to be, thanks to new and improved technology. One woman who'd expected to have to spend three or four years in braces was amazed when I told her we could have her finished in eighteen months or even sooner. Others worry they'll have to get teeth pulled, or their treatment will require big bulky bands. Thirty years ago, probably 50 percent of patients had to get teeth pulled as part of their treatment, but today it's down to about 10 percent. And the ever-improving Invisalign technology means that we can use it to correct much more complex issues than used to be the case.

I'll talk more about all these new improvements in orthodontic technology later on in the book. I hope we succeed in answering whatever questions you have, and that if you've been told that you or your child needs braces (or you can see it for yourself) you'll give us a call and come in for a visit. Your initial exam and consultation are free, and I can promise you a warm welcome.

# Chapter One

# Why Is My Child's Smile So Important?

**IF YOU ARE WEIGHING** the yes/no and now/later decisions of orthodontic care or braces, you'll be trying to decide just how important or unimportant it really is.

Some parents feel "looks aren't everything." Some think their kid should just be tough-minded about this and not overly sensitive. Some may not have had orthodontic care when they were children and think, *Hey, I turned out just fine. I have a great spouse, a good career, friends—so what's the big deal?*

But that was then. This is *now*: the age of social media.

Social shaming and bullying is a lot worse, a lot more common, and a lot more persistent than when you were a kid. Teen suicide is on the rise, and such suicides share one thing in common: shocked and bewildered parents who could not conceive of their child ending his own life. Sure, they might've noticed he was a *little* depressed. They knew he was being bullied and spending more time home, alone, not leaving his room, but geez, he *is* a teenager, after all. What once was a few days or weeks of misery contained in the cafeteria with a few bullies is now endless, expansive, and broadcast online to everybody. Behind a computer screen, it can get far nastier than most would dare in person. Sometimes, kids bully each other for no reason, being a buck-toothed girl or a boy with gaps in between their teeth is enough to exacerbate the situation.

## Signs Your Child May Be Being Bullied

- decrease in self-esteem
- not wanting to go to school
- skipping school
- injuries they can't explain
- self-destructive behaviors (e.g., harming themselves)
- declining school grades
- sleep difficulties
- loss of interest in schoolwork or activities
- sudden loss of friends or avoiding social groups
- changes in eating habits

A straight, clean and healthy smile can not only give your child the confidence she needs to embrace her true worth, but can also pave the way toward easier socialization at school, church, or during extracurricular activities. Do your child a favor and talk about her smile and how it might be affecting her.

Beyond that, there's a life ahead of your child. Going to junior high with crooked teeth and a humiliating smile is one thing. Hey, plenty of kids are going to school *without shoes* for heaven's sake. But going to college admission interviews, packing up and heading off to college, going to job interviews, trying to fit into new and anxiety-rich environments at a faraway college or new workplace with a bad smile—and maybe unavoidable bad breath with it—and daytime headaches from nighttime teeth-grinding is a lot more serious.

This isn't *just* a cosmetic issue. Misaligned, crooked teeth equal *significant* medical problems.

Poorly aligned teeth can produce chronic headaches and migraines, contribute to digestive problems because of the inability to properly chew foods, and make getting a decent night's sleep impossible. Perhaps the most dangerous of all: it can foster gum disease. Gum disease has absolute links to diabetes, heart disease, and strokes, as well as, of course, the loss of natural teeth altogether. Orthodontic corrections later in adult life are more difficult; they can be painful, require time off work, and at best, they'll just be embarrassing. *Invisible braces aren't really totally invisible, and you're thirty-eight? Forty-four? Fifty-one? C'mon.*

Uncorrected mouth problems and misaligned teeth make for strangely stretched gums inevitably destined to separate from teeth. This could allow "pockets" for infections and periodontal disease to arise and turn into *very* difficult, painful, and costly problems late in life.

In the teenage years, failure to spend even $4,000 can easily create a $40,000 full mouth restoration case at age forty or fifty, or embarrassing, health-compromising removal of all teeth and use of dentures at age sixty.

Gum disease is serious business. It worsens the risks of and heightens dangers from diabetes, heart disease and strokes. Ignoring preteen or teen teeth misalignment may virtually guarantee adult medical problems. If there is a genetic history of any of these medical problems I just named, you only worsen the odds of your son or daughter suffering from them by ignoring or postponing needed orthodontic treatment.

Aside from impacting health, a poorly aligned smile can significantly impact your child's comfort. Headaches, toothaches, sinus problems, dry mouth, snoring, drooling, and bad breath are all signs of a smile that isn't straight, jaws that aren't aligned, or teeth that are too close together or not quite close enough. Oftentimes, however, the mouth is the last place we check for signs of discomfort, loss of sleep, or even a simple headache.

If your child's pediatrician can't figure out why she's not sleeping well or experiencing headaches or even insomnia for which there seems to be no cause, a simple thirty-minute exam at your local orthodontist could provide a clear solution in no time!

Here is what I'm told by an awful lot of parents:

"I had wonderful parents, *but* I sure wish they had found a way to afford the braces I needed and gotten me the care I needed when I was a kid, so I didn't grow up to have this bad smile my whole life."

And what I hear from almost every adult patient getting orthodontic treatment and braces is:

"I had wonderful parents, *but* I sure wish they had found a way to afford the braces I needed and gotten me the care

I needed when I was a kid, so I didn't grow up to have this bad smile my whole life *and have all these problems now.*"

Is this how you want your daughter or son talking about you ten, twenty, or thirty years from now? Is this how you want them remembering their childhood? Your parenting?

If that sounds pretty pushy, I admit: it is. I kept it in the book for the very simple reason that this is *truly* what I have heard so much over the years, and I am sincere about letting you reflect on it. All parents want to do the right thing. They don't want to let their children down in any way, and I'm sure you don't either.

You know, parents just about kill themselves over their kids' college, trying their best to guide the decision, trekking around the country on campus visits, worrying over campus culture, or taking on *serious* debt. Every parent understands what many kids can't— that it's not about the few years of college but rather the forty or fifty years afterward.

I assure you, this is the same. It's not about the bad, humiliating smile and bad bite transformed now, for high school. It's about the many, many years to come. They really can't appreciate that now, but *you* can.

No parent wants their child to suffer, either from teeth that actually hurt, headaches you can't explain, or insecurity your child may be feeling because of a crooked or oversized smile. The fact is, your child's formative years are actually the most sensitive for his or her teeth. Now is the time to pay close attention to your child's smile, behavior, peer relationships, and confidence level.

If any or all are lacking, a qualified orthodontist may help give you and your child the peace of mind you both crave.

## The Top Five Reasons People Avoid Seeing the Orthodontist

1.  **Patients are afraid it's going to hurt.** Pain is the number-one reason most people avoid going to the orthodontist. However, modern technology—and choosing the right orthodontist—can ensure that your child enjoys a pain-free orthodontic experience.

2.  **Patients are afraid it's going to cost too much.** Not only are most orthodontic procedures more affordable than ever, but insurance, payment plans, and a variety of other financing options make this all but a moot point for most of my patients. Remember, orthodontists aren't in this to get rich, they're here to make sure your child's teeth, smile, and jaw are aligned to make his or her life better—period! We're not going to let something like price get in the way of creating a better, safer, healthier smile for your child.

3.  **Patients are afraid it's going to take too long / they're going to miss too much school or work.** Regardless of the type of orthodontic procedure your child needs, time is of the essence. Modern technology and ease of access allows us to work around your child's school schedule with minimal absences. After initial visits, and barring the actual procedure itself, most visits and/or adjustments are routine and can take anywhere from fifteen to forty-five minutes.

4.  **Patients do not see the need to take action.** Eroding, crooked, or unaligned smiles can take

time to happen, but the time to act is now. Orthodontic irregularities don't just heal on their own or disappear if you ignore them. Your child's smile and overall dental health are too important to ignore out of questions of pain, convenience, or even price.

5. **Patients have been treated in the past with an attitude of indifference.** Let's face it, not all doctors are created equal. Every profession has its "bad apples," and to say dentistry is the exception would be to write fiction instead of fact. There is no room for indifference when it comes to your child's healthcare. Find an orthodontic specialist that offers not only state of the art technology for your child, but state of the art service as well. Orthodontic specialists know what it's like to sit in the chair, and should provide every opportunity for patients, especially our younger patients, to feel comfortable, safe, and secure in our care.

Call us at **919-373-3656** or go to **Wilson-Ortho.com** to schedule your own Customized Smile Analysis.

# Chapter Two

# Why Do Kids Need Braces?

**ARE BRACES SOMETHING CREATED** by orthodontists to make money, like Disney and their extra-charge FastPass? Was it a conspiracy from the very start?

Then and now, there may be some overprescribing and premature prescribing by some doctors. There are bad apples in every orchard. And you know the adage: if all he's got is a hammer, everything (and everybody) looks like a nail.

But there is a very legitimate, clinically documented, and 90 percent of the time, clearly visible reason why some kids, as young as seven, *need* orthodontic treatment and care: malocclusion.

Malocclusion is mostly genetic, so if your daughter or son has it, blame their grandparents. It's a fancy-pants term for all things related to misaligned teeth—teeth growing angled, crooked, and into a too-crowded space. It can be a single tooth, a few teeth, or the whole mouth. As I said, it is mostly hereditary, and your kids didn't get to pick their parents out of a Barbie catalog. There can be other causes too, like early, premature loss of primary teeth, chronic thumb-sucking, or even an accident that seemed to leave no lasting effect at its moment in time.

If your child is suffering from any, several, or all of the following early indicators of malocclusion, consider having them addressed by an orthodontic specialist sooner rather than later:

- **Crossbites**: A crossbite occurs when the jaw deviates to one side with an improper fit of the upper and lower teeth from left to right or front to back. Crossbites can lead to worn and chipped teeth, jaw pain, and asymmetric growth of the jaws. Left untreated, the crossbite will require more extensive treatment later in life and significant jaw surgery in the most-severe cases.

- **Thumb-sucking**: Thumb-sucking habits beginning at the age of seven or older should be corrected immediately in order to prevent severe jaw and tooth alignment problems.

- **Miscellaneous concerns**: There are several associated issues you should also be looking for as soon as your child turns seven in order to intervene early, including the following:

    - permanent teeth that are growing into the wrong spots

    - severely protruded front teeth at risk for injury or causing teasing at school

    - severe crowding with permanent teeth erupting into poor-quality gum tissue

With any of these situations, we can discuss the pros and cons of early intervention and treatment versus waiting until all the permanent teeth are in for braces. If you are anxious about the appearance of your child's teeth or your child is self-conscious about his or her appearance, early treatment might be the best choice. Not only are most orthodontic problems more difficult to correct later, but self-image and personality inhibition can be hard for a person to leave behind. However, if your child is extremely resistant to braces or is not mature enough to be trusted to care for them, delay may be the better choice. In that case, regularly scheduled orthodontic checkups will be necessary.

Having malocclusion does *not* guarantee a child will need braces. Frankly, this is what worries me about nonspecialists like family dentists substituting themselves for orthodontists, and parents letting it happen. They may easily miss an early diagnosis of malocclusion, when it could have been treated without braces. Or they may leap to braces as the only way to treat all malocclusion. Either way, you and your child lose.

The first question, then, is: does your daughter or son have or show all the signs they are going to have malocclusion? Second, if so, what—of numerous options—should be done about it? Third, when?

To have all these questions answered early, the first full orthodontic exam should occur early in a child's life. I recommend seven or eight, no later than nine, especially if there is family history of malocclusion. With early and periodic exams by an orthodontic specialist, you may avoid your child's need for braces and/or you may prevent years of suffering and embarrassment related to their teeth and smile.

Waiting will have very serious consequences, often requiring more treatment and higher costs later in life. What most parents fail to realize is that these treatment problems are urgent and should be treated as such. If that ship has sailed, the next best time for a full orthodontic exam is tomorrow at three o'clock.

If your son or daughter does need braces—now or at some predictable future time—the outcome of the exam can lead to *sensible* decisions. If not now, treatment to minimize future complications can begin, and also, you can begin saving money for braces or other procedures if necessary later on in your child's life. There is no tooth fairy coming to leave a few thousand dollars underneath his pillow or yours. But if the need must be met three years from now, skipping one Starbucks run a week for those three years can make a hefty dent in the bill to come. Utilizing a Health Savings Account or Flex Spending Account can help, as well. How to fund orthodontic treatment is discussed later in the book.

Let me be emphatically clear. I am *not* in the business of putting braces on any child who doesn't need braces. My office is *not* a braces store. I'm in the business of helping kids and families get the right orthodontic treatment if any is needed, get the right braces if any are needed, and have as perfect a smile and as few oral health problems as possible. I make sure my patients are informed—that's why I wrote this book. In my office, you're never told what to do. You're provided with real information, no medical jargon, plain English, "reasons why," and options. You probably know the term "God complex," referring to a person who acts like he's God—imperious, brusque, and deliberately intimidating to squash questions. You will *not* get that kind of treatment here, from me or anyone on my team.

Kids do need braces, but not all kids and certainly not the same braces for all. Some kids are better served by other orthodontic treatments instead of or before braces. We will collaborate, you and I, to figure out what is or isn't needed and what options are best if there is a need for your child.

Call us at **919-373-3656** or go to **Wilson-Ortho.com** to schedule your own Customized Smile Analysis.

# Chapter Three

# Why Not Just a Dentist?
# Why an Orthodontist?

**YOU UNDOUBTEDLY ALREADY** have a dentist.

*Gee, isn't seeing an orthodontist going to cost a lot more?*

*I'm busy. More appointments?*

*Do I really need to get orthodontic checkups for my kids?*

Don't worry, these are all reasonable questions! It is true that, today, quite a few dentists dance over into our territory, and although they're *not* permitted to claim they're the same as orthodontists or provide orthodontic treatment (beware of any who do), they're able to do things like provide Invisalign and other braces. This can be confusing. Here are the facts.

All orthodontists are dentists and we all graduate from the same dental schools. True enough. But that's where it stops for dentists. Orthodontists go to school for an additional two to three years to become credentialed specialists at diagnosing and providing the best treatment for conditions like:

- difficulties chewing or biting
- constant biting into the cheek, gums, or roof of the mouth
- teeth that meet abnormally or don't meet at all
- teeth grinding or clenching
- crowded, misplaced, or blocked out teeth
- early or late loss of teeth
- teeth grown in badly
- teeth that protrude
- embarrassing personal appearance due to teeth
- facial imbalances
- teeth or jaw misalignment, TMJ
- chronic headaches and migraine
- speech difficulties (that may never be outgrown or may develop later)

These are *not* dental care issues. They are orthodontic issues.

For *some* things, a generalist or jack-of-all-trades will do. For other things, you know it's smart to seek out the best specialist you can afford. For example, if all your income is in a single W-2 from one employer and you have simple, ordinary deductions, getting your taxes prepared for the cheapest fee at the seasonal H&R Block office that opens up in your neighborhood shopping center is probably fine. But if you have W-2, 1099, and investment income from real estate, depreciation on real estate in several states, own stocks, and you raise iguanas as a money hobby, you're going to get yourself a really good accountant, probably a CPA. If you need the simplest will, leaving everything first to spouse or second to daughter may be okay. But if you are of some means and have several children and maybe also grandchildren as well as charities, you're going to need to see an *estate planning* attorney, not just any attorney—though they all went to the same law schools—but *a specialist in estate planning*.

This is no different.

There are a few things to keep in mind when differentiating between a general dentist and an orthodontic specialist.

First, generalists, or jacks-of-all-trades, tend to work with one-size-fits-all, off-the-rack, standardized solutions. They may be limited to doing only what the computer dictates that they do, without bringing expertise and expert judgment to bear. They're often working with products from only one provider, without being able to select from a full range of options that would work best for you. Specialists, instead, tend to individually and carefully diagnose needs and provide personalized solutions.

Second, generalists and their use of inexpertly applied, standardized solutions tend to be cheaper than the fees of a specialist, but that also places economic pressure on them to do the treatment as quickly and simply as possible, because they've "cut it thin."

In this case, it's worth remembering that the treatment provided has permanent, lifelong, and life-impacting consequences. This concerns your health, future dental or jaw alignment or misalignment issues affecting quality of sleep (which can affect weight, even onset and management of type 2 diabetes and heart disease), as well as self-esteem and social and career success.

**General Dentist.** A general dentist gives routine checkups, preventative measures, cleans teeth, and fixes cavities. They may not start seeing children until they are seven to ten years old.

**Pediatric Dentist.** A pediatric dentist has two to three years of specialized education beyond dental school. They specialize in providing dental care to children and adolescents, offering checkups, preventative measures, cleanings, and cavities.

**Orthodontist.** An orthodontist has two to three years of specialized education beyond dental school and is an expert at straightening teeth and aligning the jaws. They assess patients and determine the best treatment routes and procedures that need to be taken.

If you can, you want to choose an orthodontist for orthodontic care.

You may ask, *how do I know my doctor is an orthodontist?* It's a good question and a critical one to ask as you seek additional treatment for your child's dental issues.

Only orthodontists can belong to the American Association of Orthodontists (AAO). If you're looking for a local orthodontist, go online and visit **www.braces.org** to find a specialist in your area. This website features not only a searchable database of orthodontists but educational tips, answers and resources to help you on your quest for your child's healthiest smile!

Alternatively, you can ask your doctor if he or she has completed a two- to three-year residency in orthodontics and check with your state dental board to follow up on his reply. Dentists and orthodontists in most states will be registered differently with the dental board.

Do your homework; be a "dental detective" while on the hunt for such vital information. Look for the words "dental specialist in orthodontics," or ask your general dentist for a referral to a specialist. In urban and suburban areas, it will take minimal effort to find a specialist. In more remote, rural locations, your search might take you to another city or town. Don't be afraid to ask your dentist if an orthodontist travels to your town every month to see patients. There's a chance an orthodontist from a larger city comes to your town and works out of another dental office once or twice per month. Looking around can save valuable driving time and money.

One note: there is no disrespect between orthodontists and dentists. As a matter of fact, many orthodontic patients are referred by their dentists. These are great, capable, and caring professionals who know where their expertise begins and ends, and who do not let ego or income opportunity step in front of what they know is best for their patients. Just as the family doctor refers his patients with possible or significant heart disease issues to a cardiologist, and if need be, the cardiologist refers to a surgeon, the best dentists refer patients with orthodontic needs to orthodontists. Orthodontists are required to take two to three years of university education beyond dental school and additional continuing clinical education every year. They must also invest in state-of-the-art technology for their offices (not found in dental offices)—*all for a good reason.*

Even though we orthodontists have the education and training to perform general dentist procedures, we don't. We specialize.

Call us at **919-373-3656** or go to **Wilson-Ortho.com** to schedule your own Customized Smile Analysis.

# Chapter Four

# Choose a Highly Successful Orthodontist

**WHY IS THAT IMPORTANT?** Wouldn't you get a "better deal" from one barely getting the light bill paid? Maybe. But an overeager orthodontist—or maybe more so, an overeager dentist eager to do braces—might be seeing needs that are more urgent than they really are.

## What are some good clues to selecting a great orthodontist?

I've got two: his practice is busy.

I assure you, the ability of advertising to attract orthodontic patients is limited and it's expensive. When you see a really, really busy practice, there are probably a whole lot of patient referrals, and neither kids nor parents enthusiastically refer if they feel they were lied to or treated badly, put in pain, or wound up with results nothing like the digital future-photo they were shown. And they probably wouldn't come to that practice if they had to keep coming back to "fix a few things," or were overcharged. Parents tell parents about great orthodontic practices because we earned their trust and because their kids keep thanking them.

I keep my office very busy. Yes, we advertise. But mostly, these practices thrive by patient referrals. Not that I would anyway, but I don't need to goad you into more and more expensive care than your son's or daughter's situation requires for the best outcome. I don't need to "sell" four more sets of braces this month to win a cruise from the manufacturer—and yes, that stuff goes on in some practices. There's an old cartoon from the *Wall Street Journal* with a bunch of executives in a boardroom at a conference table, one hollering, "Ethics? Ethics? We can't afford ethics!"

This is a business, a business built on ethics and earned trust. And you do *not* just need a doctor to install braces; you need a trust-worthy advisor.

The other clue: a great orthodontist is *not* cheap.

Our fees are calculated to allow for "Cadillac + Care" in every respect, to put no downward financial pressure on how we care for patients and parents, and to *never* cut corners or take shortcuts. We *never* use any material that is "probably good enough."

If I were you, I'd worry if I could find an orthodontist that is a lot cheaper anywhere else. If you do find one, know this: behind closed doors they're probably asking, "Can we do this cheaper?" Is *that* the question you want discussed back there, at every step of your child's treatment?

This isn't even like Botox. It's more like cosmetic surgery. There's a science and an art to this. Myself and my team are all highly trained to produce state-of-the-art outcomes, nothing less. The doctor makes a difference. That's why I tell everybody to get a highly successful orthodontist.

## The Top Ten Things You Should Know *Before* Choosing Your Orthodontist

This is something you want to be sure about.

I've just suggested one big consideration: a very successful practice. Here are ten more.

### 1. Are they a specialist?

Orthodontists are specially trained dentists who take on several extra years of training in order to "straighten teeth," usually by affixing braces to the patient's teeth. You might say we specialize in smiles. Orthodontists also perform dentofacial orthopedics. This is a fancy way to describe how we normalize the structure of a patient's jawbones in order to repair any imbalance in their face. All orthodontists are dentists, but only 6 percent of dentists are orthodontists. Look for the seal of the American Association of Orthodontists (AAO). Only orthodontic specialists can belong to the AAO.

### 2. Do they treat adults?

Orthodontics is not just for kids! It's important that your orthodontist can treat patients of all ages. Many adults are finding out how a healthy and attractive smile is important to their health and the way they feel about themselves. Others choose to avoid a lifetime of crooked teeth for health concerns or problems with their bite.

## 3. Do they provide the first visit free of charge?

Most orthodontists offer free examinations for new patients so you and your family can get expert advice about treatment needs, options, and timing before making this important investment. During your first exam and consultation be sure your questions are answered, your concerns are addressed, and you are educated about all of your treatment options. The orthodontist should include digital x-rays during the exam at no charge.

## 4. Do they offer guarantees? If so, what are they?

No matter which orthodontist you choose, ultimately you are not making a small investment. That being said, wouldn't you want to ensure your orthodontist is going to stand behind their treatment? Of course! We wouldn't have it any other way. In fact, we offer a satisfaction guarantee. If your child has any issues or if you are not satisfied with the treatment, our team of smile specialists will make it right, guaranteed.

## 5. Are they using the latest technology and treatment options available?

Orthodontics today differs a great deal from years past. Computer-designed braces and wires dramatically increase the precision with which we move teeth and shorten treatment time. Tie-free braces systems have made treatment far more efficient and comfortable. Clear braces offer a cosmetically pleasing alternative, while Invisalign offers patients an entirely brace-free option. Did you know that Invisalign also has a special treatment system just for teens? Ultimately, you get the best treatment available when you choose us.

## 6. Does their quoted fee include retainers?

Each orthodontic office has its own fee schedules, and doctors often charge differently for procedures. All orthodontists should offer you a contract that clearly spells out the expenses for your child's treatment before it begins.

Throughout the orthodontic industry, it's common to find out about retainer fees after you start treatment. You should ask your orthodontist about what retainers cost and also if there are any other hidden fees.

## 7. Do they charge for emergency appointments?

Some minor discomfort may occur with braces. Orthodontists typically provide adjustments for poking wires and loose appliances free of charge. While we do provide these types of adjustments free of charge, you should definitely ask about adjustments and potential costs with your orthodontist before you start treatment.

Keep in mind that if your braces are broken or damaged due to noncompliance with dietary restrictions, this may result in repair charges. If you do your best to avoid breaking your braces and follow the simple dietary guidelines that we will share with you, then you should have no additional costs for adjustments throughout your treatment, even if it's an emergency.

## 8. Do they make you feel special and comfortable?

Regardless if you are reading this book for your own treatment or for your child's treatment, when you meet with your orthodontist, you should definitely feel comfortable. We strive to make you as comfortable as possible before, during, and after treatment. You are special and we want you to feel special every time you see us.

Particularly important if you are reading this book for the treatment of your child, we also ensure your child feels special every time they visit. Since our team is so involved with children and young adults, we can empathize, relate to them, and make them feel comfortable and extra special.

## 9. Do they have a great reputation?

With the internet, it is extremely easy to pull up ratings and reviews from patients. Simply go to Google and search for orthodontist reviews and ratings in your town.

Additionally, look on the website for video testimonials from actual patients. You can also ask the orthodontist for references.

## 10. Are they flexible with payment options?

Once you are comfortable and you know specifically which orthodontist you want to treat you or your child, the next question is typically, "How much is this going to cost and how am I going to pay for this?"

We help you understand different payment options from maximizing the most insurance benefits to flex spending accounts to even interest-free payment plans. During the initial exam and complimentary consultation, we will answer all of your questions, including those about our typical cost of braces and the variety of payment options available.

## How to Know What Questions to Ask

I've really thought through the questions most parents and patients have—not just the ones they ask, but the ones they don't. This book attempts to cover them all, but again, this is a *personal* matter. The best questions to ask are the ones that matter most to you and your child.

I hope not, but you may be in a position that absolutely requires you to get the minimum essential treatment for the lowest cost. If so, your most important questions are going to be about those kinds of options and about price, and nothing else.

If, however, you are able to make your decision about who you should trust with your child's oral health and smile by many factors, we've included a "What Is Most Important to You?" quiz from Excellence In Orthodontics on the following pages. As you'll see, there are fourteen different items to consider and rank in importance to you. Any can become the questions you ask me and my team or any other orthodontist.

Incidentally, Excellence In Orthodontics is a national organization for exceptionally successful orthodontists leading the field in both clinical and patient care and patient/parent (client) service excellence. We all subscribe to a pledge of very high standards and hold each other accountable. You can learn more at ExcellenceInOrthdontics.org.

If you have a specific question not answered anywhere in this book, or have a personal and confidential question, you can—with compete assurance of privacy and courtesy—email Info@Wilson-Ortho.com or call Dr. Michael Wilson at 919-373-3656.

There is also a FAQ section at the back of this book.

Of course, a perfect opportunity to get questions answered—yours and your son's or daughter's—is at your exam appointment.

Call us at **919-373-3656** or go to **Wilson-Ortho.com** to schedule your own Customized Smile Analysis.

# What Is Most Important to You?

**Directions**: For each **Key Item** below, rank its importance to you from 1 to 5. Then check off whether each type of provider provides that item. When you're done with all 14 Key Items, add up your rankings and review what your final score means about choosing an orthodontist.

| | Key Items to Consider<br><br>in Selecting Your Orthodontist | Rank How Important<br>Each Item Is to You<br><br>in Selecting Your Orthodontist<br>1 – Not Important,<br>5 – Very Important | Wilson<br>Orthodontics | Other<br>Provider | Other<br>Provider |
|---|---|---|---|---|---|
| | | | **Check Off If Provided** | | |
| **1** | Orthodontist and staff committed to expert, thorough diagnosis, and prescription of the best treatment plan customized for my son or daughter | 1 2 3 4 5 | ✓ | | |
| **2** | Avoiding extractions (if possible) | 1 2 3 4 5 | ✓ | | |
| **3** | Avoiding having to wear headgear with braces (if possible) | 1 2 3 4 5 | ✓ | | |
| **4** | Avoiding "metal-mouth" braces (if possible) or utilizing the new type of "invisible" braces | 1 2 3 4 5 | ✓ | | |
| **5** | Having a healthy, pleasing smile that will last a lifetime and protect optimum dental health (not just having straightened teeth) | 1 2 3 4 5 | ✓ | | |
| **6** | Pain-free treatment | 1 2 3 4 5 | ✓ | | |
| **7** | Orthodontist utilizes the most modern, advanced, and proven technology, including computer-aided design and fitting | 1 2 3 4 5 | ✓ | | |
| **8** | Orthodontists and team actively involved in continuing clinical education | 1 2 3 4 5 | ✓ | | |
| **9** | Reducing treatment time to a minimum without compromising results (including total length of treatment term and number of office visits) | 1 2 3 4 5 | ✓ | | |
| **10** | Availability of after-school or after-work appointment options | 1 2 3 4 5 | ✓ | | |
| **11** | Treatment coordinator is knowledgeable about insurance coverage and is able to offer flexible payment plans | 1 2 3 4 5 | ✓ | | |

| | | | | | | | | | |
|---|---|---|---|---|---|---|---|---|---|
| **12** | Getting the best overall value factoring in thorough diagnosis, customized care, and concern with lifetime health and well-being—not just the cheapest fee | 1 | 2 | 3 | 4 | 5 | ✓ | | |
| **13** | Lifetime guarantee | 1 | 2 | 3 | 4 | 5 | ✓ | | |
| **14** | Orthodontist and team committed to excellence in orthodontics and customer service for both patients and parents | 1 | 2 | 3 | 4 | 5 | ✓ | | |

## Total of Your Rankings

### What Your Score Means

**50-70**   There is no doubt. Wilson Orthodontics is the right choice for you and your family! It is clear that you place a high value on a comprehensive, "best" approach.

**43-49**   You are probably also going to be happiest with Wilson Orthodontics, rather than any other alternative. But this score suggests you aren't completely sure and have some unanswered questions or concerns. Your doctor and the practice's treatment coordinator want no lingering uncertainties on your part, and want to address any and every question. Don't keep anything to yourself. Please ask.

**42 or less**   Frankly, you may not value the advanced, sophisticated level of clinical care and customer service provided at Wilson Orthodontics. Cost may be much more important to you than other factors, or very basic service may be all you feel you need. It's perfectly okay. If you choose to shop around, be sure to use this checklist in evaluating other options. Remember, you do want everything right the first time, and you want error-free orthodontics at a minimum.

# Chapter Five

# What Can I Expect at the Initial Consultation and Exam?

**MANY QUESTIONS SURROUND YOUR** first visit to a new orthodontist, not the least of which is the subject of this particular chapter: *what will happen at the initial consultation?*

To answer this very common question, and perhaps several others you might not even realize you need answering yet, let me walk you through the typical first office visit, from the initial appointment forward. Your first appointment is scheduled following your initial phone call to your orthodontist's office.

1. **On arrival at the office, you will be greeted by one of our certified treatment coordinators**. She or he is fully prepared to make everything from the first appointment to an entire treatment program go smoothly for you and your child. Your treatment coordinator will manage your relationship with us, from appointment scheduling for your convenience to answering questions.

At the initial visit, your treatment coordinator will review your child's patient information and health history and/or any appearance concerns with you.

This interview and required-by-law paperwork doesn't take long. You may also be asked to view, with your son or daughter, a pre-exam video by Excellence In Orthodontics. This video makes you and, if old enough, your son or daughter truly *informed* patients. It can reduce resistance by your preteen or teen to treatment, making life easier for you.

2. **Next, your orthodontist will conduct the "Customized Smile Analysis,"** the most complete and thorough orthodontic exam, including teeth, gums, mouth, jaws, and face. Typically, safe digital x-rays are taken of the teeth and surrounding bone and of the jaw structures. An intra-oral scan of the teeth may be made.

Usually that same day, your orthodontist will present his or her "report of findings"—a "show-n-tell," in plain English (not medical jargon), of the full state of your child's teeth, gums, mouth and jaws, and a diagnosis of any present or anticipated problems that should get orthodontic treatment. If treatment should occur, your orthodontist will present recommendations and options. This will be an individualized, personalized plan of treatment, not "braces in a box, off the shelf." By this report of findings, you will know:

- what teeth or jaw misalignment or other problems exist or are developing

- what the health and appearance ramifications are of not intervening with treatment

- if braces are needed now or later and which type of braces will be best in your situation

- what the complete treatment program will consist of, such as braces, number of appointments, and average time of each office visit

- what results will be achieved at the end of treatment

3. **All your questions will be answered**. There are no dumb or embarrassing questions. Every single one of my patients has a question, simple or complex! We do *not* want you or your son or daughter just nodding, then later wondering, "What did he mean by *that?*" or saying, "I wish I'd asked about …" This is *not* one of those "I'm the doctor—trust me—just do what I say because I said so" offices. Most questions will have been answered by the pre-exam video, other literature provided to you, this book, and your orthodontist's report of findings, but it's a lot to take in. So, any and all questions you have should be asked and answered. Our goal is not just a terrific orthodontic outcome ensuring a healthy, attractive smile, but also your anxiety-free comfort from start to finish.

4. **Finally, your treatment coordinator will explain the costs of the prescribed treatment program and discuss payment arrangements as needed**. Before proceeding, the next two appointments will be scheduled for the installation of braces and/or other treatment. As the saying goes, a journey of a thousand steps begins with the first one, and a task well begun is sooner done!

In total, you should allow about one hour for this entire initial consultation and exam.

If that seems like a lot, keep in mind there are *lifetime* health, appearance, and personality aspects of this. And it's not "installing tires"—not if it's done properly and expertly. Your son or daughter deserves a careful, thorough, and anxieties-eliminated experience. You want to make the best decisions for them.

Frankly, our practice and our process is not for everybody. We attract and "resonate with" parents who are quite serious about their responsibilities and committed to giving their child every possible advantage in life—certainly not unnecessary disadvantages. If you are that parent—and the fact that you took the trouble to obtain and read this book suggests it—then you are going to recognize that this is time well invested in the best possible results.

Call us at **919-373-3656** or go to **Wilson-Ortho.com** to schedule your own Customized Smile Analysis.

*"This experience was simply AMAZING! I love how professional the staff was and how informative Dr. Wilson was each and every time we went in for a visit. I am very pleased with the treatment results we received. To see my son smile and feel confident and proud of his smile is the best feeling ever!"*

**—SHIRLEY S.**

# Chapter Six

# Shouldn't There Be a Guarantee?

**HEALTH CARE IS NOTORIOUS** for no guarantees.

Surgeons have a dark-humor insiders' joke: dead patients can't sue.

If you've seen reality TV shows about plastic surgery, like the popular one airing as I wrote this, *Botched*, you know things can go horribly wrong.

Guarantees are controversial in all kinds of health care, including orthodontics. Many doctors are upset by the very idea. One huffed and puffed at me, "What do you think you're doing with this guarantee nonsense? We aren't operating a car shop, installing mufflers and guaranteeing them for five thousand miles. We are doctors, dammit."

His ego was mightily offended. But I doubt you will be, with the challenge of deciding who should be your family's *trusted* orthodontist. So, yes, I think there should be a guarantee! In fact, many guarantees!

1.  **If you aren't satisfied with your son or daughter's orthodontic treatment, new smile outcome, or patient/ parent experience,** *our team of specialists will make it right, guaranteed.*

2.  **Also, the quality of the orthodontic treatment itself is** *guaranteed for life*. If ever the proper teeth alignment originally achieved somehow begins to fail, we will welcome you back and do everything we can to correct the problem.

3.  **You also have a safety in numbers guarantee.** The diagnostic and prescriptive methods and state-of-the-art technology and the braces products we use have been used by top orthodontists nationwide to treat over one million patients successfully.

4.  **You also have my guarantee that** *every* **orthodontic assistant at my office and I have not only been academically educated but also** *thoroughly* **trained.** All patient care is supervised and reviewed by me. We also invest in frequent state-of-art clinical continuing education for our team exceeding all state licensing requirements. Above and beyond.

5.  You also have *my guarantee of exceptional courtesy and customer service*. Yes, you are my patient, but we can be honest about this—my practice is not just a health care provider, it is a *business*. As such, it has, in my opinion, one set of responsibilities to you as the parent of a patient and one set to the patient, including telling the whole truth and nothing but the truth, prescribing in the patient's best interest, and delivering the best possible treatment and outcomes. There's also a second, separate set

of responsibilities to you as a customer, including access, convenience, responsiveness, and "red carpet service."

These five guarantees are included in your treatment program fee.

For starters, I can guarantee you the best, most thorough orthodontic exam, and I encourage coming in for it now.

Call us at **919-373-3656** or go to **Wilson-Ortho.com** to schedule your own Customized Smile Analysis.

# Chapter Seven

# How to Get More Information

**THERE ARE SEVERAL WAYS** to get information about an orthodontic practice. First, I want to address the ways I don't recommend.

I don't recommend Yelp. Yelp is, unfortunately, not at all what it seems, and is frequently the subject of lawsuits from business owners, under regulatory scrutiny centered around the poorly policed manipulation of reviews, and has even been accused of the flooding of fake reviews—by "bots" no less! Some companies can use Yelp as competitive warfare while other companies turn around and sell the business owner under negative-review-assault "reputation management services." So, beware! Get the information you need from truly trusted sources.

Google can also be deceptive, though I admit it can be a valuable starting point. Rankings are manipulated by advertisements, websites, YouTube content, and what's called SEO, or search engine optimization. The only thing you know for sure about dentists or orthodontists who come up at the top in Google rankings in your community is that they are good at SEO or, more likely, good at paying somebody who is good at SEO. They're willing to spend money and willing to create a lot of content. Does that equate to certainty of the best diagnostic expertise, treatment, patient care, and customer service? Sometimes. Sometimes not.

So, first, the best thing to do is make certain you get all your questions answered by the orthodontist and the practice's treatment coordinator. Don't hold back. Put them on the spot. Be assertive. Don't feel you have to be deferential to the doctor! My own goal in this is to have every patient and every patient's parent *fully* knowledgeable about every aspect of the treatment so that they have *zero* anxiety.

Second, visit ExcellenceInOrthodontics.org. This is an organization of carefully chosen orthodontists joined together to provide carefully curated, vetted, authoritative, accurate, and understandable patient and parent information, hence its name. This can definitely help you decide on the questions you want answers to.

Finally, if you have a quick follow-up visit scheduled, these are wonderful opportunities to either ask questions you may have missed the first time, or to get further details from your orthodontist directly.

Now that we know where to get your most burning orthodontic questions answered, here are some simple tips I've amassed over the years to help you easily and effectively get the information you need:

## How to Get Your Questions Answered

**Make a list**. The easiest way to get what you want is to know it in advance. Make a list of the various questions you have when they arise so you can quickly and easily go down the list to assure you've got the right answers for the right questions.

**Bring it with you**. Take the list with you when you go for your child's orthodontist visit. This way you have the questions at hand at the right place at the right time. If you're calling in to get answers, you can also have the list ready and tick off one question for every answer you receive.

**Record the answers**. If your orthodontist, or their receptionist, speaks too fast or you can't keep up while writing the answers down, why not record them? Your cell phone likely has a "record" feature, and if not, there are many affordable micro-recorders on the market today.

**Double-check**. Finally, make sure you have the right answer by double-checking with your orthodontist or their receptionist or assistant.

Knowing where to find the information you need is only half the battle; follow these tips and you'll know how to get what you're looking for as well.

Regardless of how many questions you have, or your comfort level with technology, phone calls, or in-person visits, your orthodontist should offer an option that fits your schedule and makes all your unresolved issues crystal clear.

Call us at **919-373-3656** or go to **Wilson-Ortho.com** to schedule your own Customized Smile Analysis.

# Chapter Eight

# How to Pay For Orthodontic Treatment and Braces

**YOU MAY HAVE NEVER** needed braces. Or you may have needed them and gotten them. Or you may be among the tens of thousands of people in our generation who needed them but did not get them, perhaps because your family decided they couldn't afford them. Maybe they didn't consider it a priority and probably underestimated the lifelong results of the decision. You may not only have lived with a "hide your smile" habit unnecessarily, but you may have developed chronic jaw pain and headaches, difficulty chewing, or even periodontal disease that could have been prevented.

Regardless of which group you're in—and I hope it's not the third—I hope you will be making the best choices for your son or daughter today, without being hamstrung just by the finances. Truth is, parents pay out the same cost for a number of different things not nearly as vital as health or emotional well-being without blinking, mostly because it's paid in installments or just never really *considered,* like the monthly cost for minutes/data on mobile devices, added up for a year or two. The additional insurance cost and other costs when the teenager gets his driver's permit; after all, what's the choice? The cost of braces leaps up and stands there, all at one time. So, it can seem big. And it tempts thoughts of, "maybe later," or, "is this really necessary?"

I hope in the prior chapters I have succeeded at getting the "is it really necessary?" question erased. If there is visible need or if expert examination by an orthodontist and his explanation of what he finds can show you say it is advisable, it *is* necessary! It won't fix itself. It will probably get worse. It plagues a person's health, emotional well-being, social life, and career. It can link to very serious medical problems. *Necessary* is not really debatable.

Now let's tackle the ugly matter of the money.

I say "ugly" because nobody really likes talking about this. Most orthodontists are nervous about it. Parents are uncomfortable with it. If there is a financial obstacle to treatment, most people are reluctant to admit it, offer other excuses, and then can't be helped by the doctor. I think we have to trust each other. With me, this discussion is entirely confidential, in a "safe zone." Orthodontists are not Martians, by the way; *we* have kids, college tuitions that loom, and family budgets.

## What Is a Reasonable Fee and Cost?

A complete treatment program, including braces, can cost anywhere from $4,000 to $10,000 or so. Most fall in between. Adjusted for inflation, these prices are actually *less than* braces decades ago, while the technology and quality has advanced. In costs it can prevent later, it's a bona fide bargain. TMJ treatments are expensive. Cosmetic dentistry work is expensive. Migraine headache drugs are expensive and have side effects.

For this investment, you will be getting the carefully selected, personalized solution to your child's irregularities and problems, prescribed using state-of-the-art digital technology along with the expertise of a specialist, and considerate, compassionate care from start to finish. Your investment includes a varying number of appointments plus the orthodontic appliance itself, after-care, and in my office, certain guarantees.

It's hard to really draw a fair comparison, but if you have any significant net worth, you can easily pay similar fees for the services of an attorney expert in estate planning. Most kitchen remodels cost considerably more. Where real expertise is involved and the stakes of getting it wrong are high, you can't escape professional level fees.

In this case, the $4,000 to $10,000 range is seen as perfectly reasonable by the overwhelming majority of parents that I talk to. Each year, we provide braces of one kind or another to countless patients. Even parents who shook their heads at the cost to start with tell me afterward that having witnessed everything we do to get the absolute best obtainable results, and seeing the outcome itself, they feel undercharged.

While it's never easy to part with such a sum, people do it every day for all sorts of less important things, like their new designer handbag, golf vacation, or suite of living room furniture. They'll pay for it outright or with their favorite credit card (getting the reward points in the bargain). If you put the orthodontic treatment program including braces on a typical credit card at the interest in play as I write this, and you choose to make only the minimum required monthly payment, your monthly payments will be relatively small.

Even tight budgets can accommodate this *when it is really important.* It's less than most families pay for their cable and streaming entertainment. For many, if they got all their Starbucks stops consolidated into one monthly bill, it would be more than this!

## Health Spending Accounts (HSA) / Flex Spending Accounts (FSA)

The HSA allows you to set aside *pre-tax* dollars to be used for certain medical and health expenses for you or your family. They exist although restricted under the Affordable Care Act (Obamacare) as it stood in July of 2017. By the time you read this, the opportunity may have been expanded, as President Trump suggested. In any case, if you have accumulated money in an HSA, you can probably spend it on orthodontic treatment. If you don't have an HSA, you might want to start one. Information can be found online about existing or new accounts and their rules of use, at www.healthcare.gov.

Other kinds of FSAs are typically set up through your place of employment and similarly enable you to set aside pre-tax dollars for medical expenses. Sometimes, employers match contributions. Again, you can almost certainly tap funds from your FSA for your child's orthodontic care. Check with your employer about this.

If you have a tax accountant, you may want to consult with him about your HSA or FSA.

**TIP**: How can you make the most out of your employer's flex-pay plan? First, make sure you understand how it works. Second, set aside flex-spending dollars in advance of need, and if possible, make the maximum contributions. Many employers allow higher limits than you'd think without asking, as much as $2,500 to $5,000 per year. Be aware of "family status changes" allowed by your plan that may enable you to change the amount being moved pre-tax from your paychecks to your account anytime during the year rather than just once at the first of the year—so you could bump up the amount in months before the first orthodontic treatment. IMPORTANT: be aware of the balance and the loss of unused funds. In most cases, if you do not use these funds, you lose them, year to year. You usually have three months after the end of the calendar year to submit claims for eligible expenses from the previous year.

## Insurance

These days, there are as many different types of insurance plans as there are patients in my office. I can't possibly speak to your unique and personal insurance policy without seeing it first but, in general, my experience tells me that "most" insurance policies cover "some" of your orthodontic expenses.

I realize that answer sounds very vague, but here are a couple of variables you need to answer before an insurance agent can help you determine what, how long, and how many procedures fall under your insurance:

- the type of procedure (braces, Invisalign, etc.)

- the duration of the procedure (two months, six months, a year, etc.)

- the cause of the procedure (a patient presenting with pain, a parent's concern, traumatic injury or accident, congenital birth defect like cleft lip or palate, etc.)

- the nature of the procedure (to correct pain/discomfort, cosmetic, etc.)

I can only partially answer this question, but talking to your insurance agent will help you get the right answers you need.

**TIP**: Keep an insurance journal of every interaction with your carrier. Write down the date, time of call, name of the person you contacted, and the exact instructions or recommendations following the call. Later, if your insurance company doesn't remember what they told you, you'll have it accurately written down. If they still don't remember, ask them to pull the recorded audio tape from your previous call, so that you can accurately "remind" them of exactly what they told you.

## Loans

If you qualify, we offer Care Credit, which can provide an unsecured, signature-only loan for the treatment program, with repayment over twelve to sixty months. You don't need to go anywhere else to apply or do paperwork; we can take care of it in my office.

If you have equity in your home, the lowest-cost loan option may be a home equity line of credit or second mortgage. See your own bank, or check out RocketMortgage at rocket.quickenloans.com. As of this writing, mortgage interest is at record lows.

Obviously, a private loan from a family member can be the easiest option. A lot of preteens' and teens' important orthodontic care is financed at the Bank of Grandma and Grandpa.

If the other options are difficult or unavailable, we will set up a weekly, bimonthly, or monthly "paycheck payment plan" with a comfortable monthly payment. In the majority of situations, a down payment can be made, and the remaining balance can be paid—interest free—over the course of eighteen to twenty-four months.

## What If You Really, Really Can't Afford Braces?

I have compiled a list of eighteen ways you may be able to substantially reduce the cost of braces. Frankly, some of them are less than ideal, and most are not available through my office, but they could be helpful if your back is really up against a financial wall.

1. **Get braces in April or November and see if you can save a little extra by paying in full.** These are the months that orthodontists are the least busy, and it's when we have our most meetings (April–May). In November, everyone is getting ready for the holidays or the office is closed the week of Thanksgiving. By scheduling during the "off season," you can often find better deals with willing orthodontists.

2. **See if you can get a discount for not breaking any brackets.** Believe it or not, most orthodontists would happily take $100 off your final bill if you don't break any appliances throughout treatment!

3. **New technology; better pricing.** See if you can be one of your orthodontist's first patients with a new technology and save some money on the lab fee or receive a discount for being a teaching case.

4. **See if your local dental school has an orthodontic program.** The treatment at such institutions is supervised by board-certified orthodontists (most of whom practice in the surrounding area). While you might spend a little more time in the chair as a teaching case, if you have the time, it might be well worth the wait because you can save up to *half the cost of traditional braces.*

5. **Ask your insurance plans when they send out their fee schedules to participating providers.** If the insurance company updates their fees or the orthodontist raises his or her fees to keep up with the cost of inflation, it might be around November in preparation for the next year.

6. **See your dentist every four to six months.** While you're wearing your braces, the extra cleaning each year can prevent tooth decay, a costly item to repair.

7. **Get your flex spending dollars in order with your employer.** If you set money aside in a flex plan, it may be "tax-free," but it comes with some stipulations: namely, you have to use it before the end of the year or else you lose it.

8. **See if you can get a second set of retainers from your orthodontist at the end of treatment.** Sometimes getting two sets of retainers at the same time can be cheaper than buying a second set later in life when you lose or break your first set.

9. **See if your husband or wife has an insurance plan that covers braces.** Be sure to enroll in the plan with enough time to spare before your child needs braces, so that the procedure is not denied by your insurance company due to a waiting period.

10. **Ask for flexible financing options.** When you boil it down to the basics, your orthodontist really just wants to help you. Regardless of his specialty, your doctor spent way too much time in school *not* to love what he does (did I mention I had to go to school for ten years to become an orthodontist?). If you're easy to work with, keep your teeth clean, and avoid breaking your braces while you're wearing them, he or she will probably be thrilled to help you finance the care, or find another way to afford the investment.

11. **Do you have multiple kids in treatment?** If so, take advantage of that fact and see if you can get a family discount. In our office, we have the Wilson Orthodontics Family Care Plan that offers discounts for multiple family members in treatment.

12. **If finances are extremely tight, you should check out the organizations that orthodontists have created to help provide pro-bono care, such as Smiles Change Lives.** There are even more foundations like this if you

have a cleft palate or other facial anomalies, like the Rheam Foundation for Cleft and Craniofacial Research.

13. **School auctions, churches, or public service entities will often receive donations from local orthodontists wishing to donate a case to the school or organization for a fundraiser.** Checking around local school newsletters or church bulletins for their upcoming silent auctions could be a great find! If you're unwilling to leave such things to chance, call your local schools or churches and ask them specifically if they have such a fund and, if so, how to apply/qualify.

14. **If you're thinking about a career change, apply at your local orthodontist's office.** Most orthodontists offer free braces to their staff and their children as an employee benefit! (And you never know, you could love your career *and* your child's new braces!)

15. **Military personnel, schoolteachers, and firefighters sometimes receive special courtesies in dental and orthodontic offices throughout the year.** Keep your ears open and you might save a few bucks or at least get a donation from the orthodontist to your organization.

16. **This tactic won't save you any money, but it could earn your organization or business some money if you have a newsletter, sports team, fund-raiser, or special event that needs a sponsor.** Ask your orthodontist. Most orthodontic offices are huge supporters of the communities in which they practice and would probably love to advertise with your organization.

17. **Got taxes?** Good! Why not use your tax refund to help pay for treatment in full and ask for a courtesy on the average fees associated with financing a full orthodontic case? In some areas, you can save as much as 10 percent on the cost of braces by simply saving your pennies and paying the entire bill at once, up front.

18. **Ask for more flexible financing through a third-party credit company like Chase Healthcare Advance, through CareCredit, or by using in-house financing through your orthodontist.** Most orthodontists will accept a reasonable down payment and split the remaining amount into easy monthly payments for your convenience. With automated withdrawals from a checking or savings account, you might be able to stretch the monthly payments out over a longer period to make each payment lower. Just don't be shocked if your orthodontist asks you to approve a credit check. A little homework up front can be well worth the effort when your monthly orthodontic bill is lower than your cell phone bill!

There's no doubt about it; braces can be expensive. However, now that you're armed with these eighteen massive, budget-saving tips, you won't need to decide between braces and your budget ever again!

Call us at **919-373-3656** or go to **Wilson-Ortho.com** to schedule your own Customized Smile Analysis.

# Chapter Nine

# What Are the Treatment Options?

**IF YOUR CHILD IS** ready for orthodontic care, one of the first discussions to have with your orthodontist is which procedure is right for him or her; there might be more options than you had ever imagined.

If you're like most people, you associate orthodontists with braces, but these days, that is just one arm of what I or any orthodontist does. Here are some of the services most orthodontists will provide their patients with during the course of routine treatment:

- metal, tie-free braces
- computer designed, custom appliances and wires made uniquely for each patient
- Invisalign clear removable aligners
- clear braces
- expanders to match jaw size and tooth size

- habit appliances to eliminate thumb sucking

- space maintainers

- retainers to prevent crowding and shifting of teeth

- facemask to help correct jaw alignment

- functional appliances to help improve facial balance

- early treatment and growth modification

- lingual braces placed behind your teeth

While many of these services may seem self-explanatory to you, several will probably not. In the following pages, I will try to elaborate on several of them, including:

- crossbite correction

- metal braces

- clear braces

- Invisalign

## Crossbite Correction

As your child's teeth begin to grow in, there's a *lot* more at work than mere gum lines, tooth fairies, and molar size. How the jaw is shaped, when it develops, and even how "normally" it develops can all affect the placement and comfort of your child's teeth.

When the upper and lower teeth grow at different rates, or even when the lower jaw grows disproportionately with the upper jaw, something known as a "crossbite" can occur.

Your child might have a crossbite if, for instance, the lower jaw is out of line with the upper jaw (kind of like a box that won't close right because one of the hinges is bent).

Or perhaps on the right side of your child's mouth, the lower teeth "stick out" a little farther than the top teeth, making the upper teeth on that side overlap in turn.

Or maybe your child's upper and lower jaws are out of alignment so instead of the top and bottom front teeth meeting "naturally" as they should, the front teeth fall somewhat behind the lower teeth. This would be the reverse of an overbite.

As you might imagine, any or all of these developments can lead to short- and long-term discomfort for your child.

### How, When, and Why Crossbites Form

You might be amazed to find out how many ways a crossbite can form as your child grows and develops during his or her formative years. Heredity is one key to jaw growth, or alignment, as is the size of your child's developing jaw.

Another factor that can contribute to the development of a potential crossbite is if it takes your child too long to lose his or her baby teeth. In some extreme cases, in fact, if it takes too long for your child to lose his baby teeth, another set of teeth can grow in behind them, throwing the alignment off and contributing to a crossbite.

Believe it or not, something as basic as whether your child breathes through her nose or her mouth can also contribute to a crossbite. While most children breathe through their noses, some children develop a habit early on of breathing through their mouths instead.

In children who breathe through their noses while they're sleeping, the tongue naturally rests on the roof of the mouth, promoting natural and proper upper jaw growth. When young children breathe through their mouths, however, the tongue relocates from the roof of the mouth to the bottom, removing that extra support and potentially contributing to reduced upper jaw bone growth; this can create the crossbite we spoke of previously.

## How Can I Spot a Crossbite?

Although it sounds severe, and even painful from the description provide earlier, the effects of a crossbite can take time to manifest themselves. Still, here are some of the telltale signs your child might be cultivating, or already suffering from, a crossbite:

- snoring
- difficulty breathing
- chewing on one side of the mouth or the other
- signs of an underbite
- if your child's chin seems "off center" or disproportionate

## How, When, and Why to Correct a Crossbite

Where should you start looking for treatment if you're concerned about your child's jaw development after reading this section? If you suspect your child might have a crossbite, approach your family dentist about a recommendation for a specialist such as an orthodontist.

There are many possible treatments available for a crossbite, and your orthodontist can work with you closely to make the right and specific decisions for you and your child.

When should you start? I believe you know my standard answer when it comes to questions like this one: *as early as possible*! The same way an auto mechanic would tell you to take care of that oil leak, bulging tire, or faulty timing belt sooner rather than later, myself and my colleagues in orthodontics will always favor early treatment to later.

Crossbites are often closely linked with other orthodontic issues, such as teeth alignment, jaw size, and growth, so naturally, the sooner you address any or all of these issues, the better.

Finally, why should you address a crossbite? Crossbites can lead to pain, discomfort, and a lack of confidence as your child begins to feel insecure or even ostracized because of this very treatable, very normal series of jaw and teeth developments.

Not only can crossbites become physically uncomfortable if left untreated, but if the misalignment or root cause of the bite isn't fixed early in childhood, then the child's appearance and, ultimately, confidence could be affected as the crossbite becomes more pronounced in adolescence.

## Metal Braces

The fact is, metal braces still have a valued place in the orthodontic world, and despite advances and breakthroughs of products like Invisalign and even clear braces, they aren't going extinct anytime soon! This is because metal braces are very strong and can withstand most types of treatment. Today's metal braces are smaller, sleeker, and more polished than ever before.

*"We have being going to Dr. Wilson for years with our oldest and now the youngest. My youngest son got his braces up top yesterday and the staff were phenomenal with him. Everything was thoroughly explained before and while putting his braces on—it made a world of difference with his anxiety. We would encourage everyone to go with Wilson Orthodontics."*

**—MICHELLE M.**

Older, traditional metal braces require an elastic o-shaped rubber band, called a ligature, to hold the arch wire onto the bracket. These elastic ties collect more plaque and bacteria, making it harder for patients to clean the teeth and gums.

You may have heard of "Damon braces" or "Speed braces." These are sometimes also referred to as "self-ligating brackets" or "tie-free braces." Self-ligating means that the brackets do not need the little o-shaped rubber bands (ligatures) or metal tie wires to hold the arch wire onto the bracket. Several companies have developed braces for holding the wires in place without ligatures.

By using self-ligation technology, the brackets allow the wire to slide back and forth. This advancement allows for fewer adjustments and fewer appointments. These types of braces do not need rubber bands to hold the arch wire in place. They use a "door" to secure the arch wire to the bracket. They're smaller than traditional metal and less food gets trapped around them when you eat.

Naturally, orthodontists are very excited about the hygiene benefits of these self-closing or tie-free metal braces. Patients are excited that their braces are small, smooth, and friction-free, and will straighten their teeth in fewer visits with less discomfort than braces with wires that are "tied-in."

## Clear Braces

Ceramic braces are very strong and generally do not stain. Two popular brands are Damon Clear, made by Ormco, and Clarity, made by 3M Unitek. Adults like to choose ceramic because they "blend in" with the teeth and are less noticeable than metal. These are the type of braces actor Tom Cruise had.

Older types of ceramic braces required white or clear ligatures (tiny rubber bands) to hold the wire on to the braces. Damon Clear is a revolutionary tie-free ceramic braces system that combines the same efficient tooth movement with exceptional aesthetics. Patients choosing Damon Clear no longer have to decide between metal braces or clear braces that could stain.

Today's clear Damon Clear braces are very aesthetic because they no longer require the small rubber bands that could stain with certain foods or drinks.

### Adult Orthodontics

It's not uncommon for individuals who have undergone orthodontic treatment earlier in life to find their teeth have drifted out of alignment over the years. Most adults won't think twice about bleaching their teeth to roll back the effects of time. Yet few think about the role orthodontics can play.

Adults of all ages can enjoy the same cosmetic and health benefits of properly aligned teeth with appliances like the Damon Clear system braces.

Improperly aligned teeth can do more than undermine your confidence. They can make proper cleaning and brushing more difficult, contribute to enamel loss, and even set the stage for more significant problems down the road. Fortunately, discrete treatment with Damon Clear braces can help keep you aligned with a healthy, happy lifestyle.

### The Solution Is Clear

Orthodontists believe every individual has the right to live their life with a smile they truly love, particularly children. Healthy, straight, and attractive smiles make your child happier and more self-confident. And isn't that what we all want for them?

Damon Clear helps you achieve the smile of your dreams faster, easier, and more discretely than you ever imagined. Embrace the confidence that comes with beautifully aligned teeth and put your smile on display. Schedule a consultation and ask if Damon Clear system braces are right for you.

The Damon Clear system uses a free-sliding technology that places almost no pressure on your teeth as it gently corrects their alignment. Less pressure means a more comfortable treatment.

With Damon Clear free-sliding braces, your treatment can proceed faster with fewer follow-up visits than traditional fixed wire braces.

## Invisalign

Invisalign is a widely advertised, well-known, and popular braces product, and kids often know about it and ask parents and doctors for it by name. For many, it's as good an option as any other and sometimes even the best option.

Invisalign uses advanced, proprietary 3-D computer-imaging technology to "map" the entire span of treatment, from the present teeth alignment to the desired positioning, alignment, and smile. Clear aligners are custom made and based on the 3-D imaging. Invisalign has many features that have helped make it such a popular choice. The aligners are removable, even before a snack or meal as well as for general hygiene. There are no metal brackets or wires. Office visits for adjustments throughout the treatment program are fast, easy and painless. The thermoplastic aligners are virtually invisible. Over one million patients have been treated with Invisalign, and there is a special Invisalign system for teens.

Because Invisalign is computer mapped, there's sometimes the idea that anybody can install Invisalign and that all practitioners using Invisalign are the same. I have an important warning about this: during each stage of the complete treatment, only certain teeth are allowed to move. Which teeth move in what order, and the amount of time (days/weeks) needed for each successive set of aligners differs for each patient. *This* is what you rely on an expert orthodontist specializing in pediatric and juvenile care to decide. At the start, we determine whether your son or daughter is a good candidate for the Invisalign approach, or if they would be better served with different braces. You have to rely on *somebody* to tell you. I promise you, there are kids who've been hurried to Invisalign who were not good candidates for it.

### Invisalign Teen

Much like the standard adult version, the Invisalign Teen System lets you do it the modern, hygienic way. Your new smile is created with the most innovative technology—a series of clear aligners that are custom-fit to your teeth.

The first thing you should know is that an average treatment takes about twelve to eighteen months. Plus, your treatment can begin even if you don't have all of your permanent teeth. Invisalign Teen was designed to meet your needs.

Invisalign Teen aligners will snap on your child's teeth easily. They are comfortable and practically invisible. Invisalign Teen allows for permanent teeth to grow gently while continuously moving teeth in small increments. Aligners are worn for about one week and then swapped for a new pair.

Invisalign Teen aligners have a "Blue Dot Wear Indicator," designed to show an estimation of wear time. The dot is designed to fade until it's clear over a one week period if you wear your aligners properly (meaning for twenty to twenty-two hours every day).

Invisalign Teen is designed to custom-fit to your child's teeth and go with his or her lifestyle. During your treatment, your child can keep smiling, playing sports, eating what he or she wants, and brushing and flossing normally because the aligners are removable. Plus, unlike traditional braces, the aligners are made of smooth plastic and move teeth gradually.

The aligners are replaceable if lost. That's right; you get up to six free individual aligners.

After your child's Invisalign Teen treatment, you may find his or her self-confidence boosted by their new smile and the change in their appearance. Some people even feel that way during the treatment. As you know, smiling has many benefits. It can help your child make a strong impression in lots of different social situations—at school, at work, or at a party.

Invisalign Teen really works. It helps correct a broad range of dental and orthodontic issues. You can get a confident smile without metal bands, brackets, or wires. It works on many kinds of conditions, including overly crowded or widely spaced teeth, crossbites, overbites, and underbites.

We've used Invisalign to successfully transform the smiles of many patients, but we do not prescribe it to everybody. After all, *popularity* should not govern medical care!

## Customizing Your Treatment

**SureSmile** is a technology that is used to fine-tune and customize your treatment to maximize effectiveness and cut down on treatment duration. First, braces are placed and the initial straightening is done as usual for the first few months. Midway through treatment the teeth are scanned into a computer to make a 3-D model of the teeth. This allows the orthodontist to design a customized set of wires for the patient that's specific to their needs. The wire is fabricated by a robot in Dallas, using a copper-nickel-titanium material that's gentler and more flexible than the rigid stainless steel material that braces were typically made of in the past. By customizing the process, it allows us to treat the patient 30 percent faster than in the past. With conventional orthodontics, the orthodontist would adjust the pressure on the patient's teeth by bending wires, seeing what happened, then adjusting those wires again. Now, this method allows us to shave significant time off the treatment, meaning that we get the desired results in eighteen months rather than over two years, and what would previously have taken eighteen months to accomplish can now be done in fourteen. Not only are you saving time, you're making fewer trips to the orthodontist's office, which is definitely a good thing.

If you've been told in the past that you were a candidate for jaw surgery to treat your crossbite, or that you'd need extractions to ease crowding in your mouth—or that there was really nothing that could be done for your case at all—it's a good idea to take advantage of the free exam and consultation an orthodontist can offer and find out what's available to you now. We can do so much more than ever before.

## Better Imaging, Better Care

For our imaging, we use what's called an i-Cat, which is a cone beam scanner that allows us to take 3-D images of the teeth. Basically, it works like a 3-D x-ray, and not only can we see much more happening with their teeth than the old 2-D x-rays revealed, we can also get a better view of how the patient's jaw is growing.

The process is very easy and more comfortable for the patient than the older x-rays were. The patient sits down, and the scanner apparatus circles their head. It literally takes seconds, and we can pull the image up on the computer immediately. I always joke that I'm turning the patient's teeth into a video game, because I can take that model on the computer screen, rotate it, segment it and look at it from the inside like I'm standing on the tongue, then look at cross-sections. It's a fantastic diagnostic tool that lets us discover things like extra teeth we wouldn't have seen previously. Sometimes, on a 2-D x-ray, an extra tooth will be overlapped so you can't really make it out, but it's revealed on the cross sections of the 3-D scan. We also get a clearer view of the roots of the teeth, which can reveal any anomalies or abnormalities. It can even be used to measure a patient's airways, which can relate to breathing issues and sleep apnea, and can help determine if a patient might need a referral to an ear, nose, and throat doctor or a sleep study if they're reporting sleep issues.

## No More Impressions?

Another great thing technology has done is eliminating the old-fashioned tray full of goop we used to have to employ to make the impressions required for Invisalign or other appliances. For Invisalign, patients would have this awkward tray in their mouths for five minutes, and nobody liked it. Sometimes we'd have to do multiple impressions before we got one that was clear. Even then, sometimes the Invisalign lab would call us and say, "Hey, that impression wasn't good. Can you take another one?" We'd have to call the patient back, which is a big inconvenience.

Now, with intraoral scanners, such as the iTero, we can use a handheld device to scan or take pictures of your teeth in under ten minutes. These images are used to make a virtual model of your teeth used for computer software simulations to determine your best treatment options. They can also be used to 3-D print aligners or other appliances.

## Trustworthy, Objective Advice

Our office is *not* "in the pocket of" or obligated to any of these providers of different braces products and technologies. We select and recommend what we believe is *the* most appropriate and beneficial choice for your child. We are happy to discuss the pros and cons of different ones, if your child has heart set on, say, Invisalign, because that's what a friend has, or based on information you've obtained.

Candidly, these manufacturers vary in price to the orthodontist (or dentist) based on volume purchase benchmarks, incentivizing concentration of as much use as possible to one product. Awards are given out to the highest volume buyers and users. It's borderline unseemly. It introduces temptation into the diagnostic and prescriptive process, and I never let us bow to such incentives and temptations. The number-one rule here is: what is absolutely best for the patient?

Call us at **919-373-3656** or go to **Wilson-Ortho.com** to schedule your own Customized Smile Analysis.

# Chapter Ten

# How Difficult Is Living with Braces

**REMEMBER, THIS ISN'T 1982.** Or 1992. Today's braces aren't anything like yours if you had them decades ago. Today's orthodontic care is far more advanced, more sophisticated, and more patient-centered than any prior generation has experienced. If you had traditional metal braces twenty years or so ago, you experienced medieval torture. The dungeon is gone too, replaced by ultra-modern, comfortable, and patient-friendly offices. Out of the dark, into the light!

Living with braces is *not* going to be anywhere near as difficult as you might imagine.

Let's look at a few specific concerns.

## Brushing and Hygiene

Modern braces, whether they're metal, flexible, or "invisible," are all actually made to fit the individual and facilitate easy, painless, thorough brushing. This means your child brushes pretty much the same as he would if he didn't have braces.

Here are some simple tips you can share with your child for the best results when brushing with braces on:

- Brush your teeth with a soft nylon toothbrush after you eat and before bed (no electric toothbrushes).[2]

- Brush, rinse, and look; if you find any areas that are not clean, brush them again.

- Brush your gums as you brush your teeth (massage and stimulate).

- Take extra care in the area between the gums and the braces because food caught and left there can cause swollen gums, cavities, discomfort, and permanent teeth stains.

- If no toothpaste is available, brush without.

- If you are unable to brush, rinse your mouth vigorously with water.

- Replace your old toothbrush when it gets worn out.

- It's absolutely essential you continue regular visits to your family dentist for checkups and cleanings throughout your orthodontic treatment!

---

2    At my office, you'll be provided with a home kit including the best toothbrush, toothpaste, and rinse.

Depending on the age of your child, you, the parent, may need to supervise the first few brushings with the braces in place. You should *not* have a whining, resistant, difficult child on your hands because of any of this. It should be painless, simple, and routine.

## Forbidden Foods Your Child Must Avoid

After your child's orthodontic appliance/braces have been placed, the teeth are usually "tender" and sensitive for as few as three to as many as ten days: a *short* time. During these few days, softer foods are recommended: soups, macaroni, spaghetti, eggs, fish, Jell-O, yogurt. As needed, Tylenol or Advil are adequate in relieving any discomfort, taken an hour or so before eating.[3] Warm saltwater rinses can be helpful. We also provide a "soft white wax," a safe topical that eases gum discomfort.

For the entire duration of the braces being in place, I'd advise you to stay away from hard and sticky foods that can damage braces and may lengthen the time they have to be worn or even require extra office visits. Sugar-rich foods can make hygiene harder and cause calculus build-up and cavities. You're probably already monitoring and limiting your child's intake of such foods, so there's really nothing new under the sun here. But, for the record, here are the "featured items" that should be avoided during orthodontic treatment and wearing of braces:

---

3    Prescription pain pills with dangerous side effects are not needed. Any orthodontist or dentist easily prescribing such drugs is not to be trusted. As you are no doubt aware from the news, opioid addiction is rampant. Pain drugs are, contrary to early assertions by their manufacturers, proving to be extremely addictive for many people after nominal and legitimate use. I can't emphasize enough—we practice truly pain-free orthodontics.

1. **Rock-hard foods**: ice (don't chew ice!), nuts, popcorn (has hard kernels inside), peanut brittle, rock candy, whole apples and carrots (unless cut into bite sized pieces), corn on the cob, hard pretzels, hard rolls, hard taco shells.

2. **Extra-sticky foods**: Jolly Ranchers or Starbursts or similar candies, bubble gum, taffy, and sticky Cinnabon rolls.

3. **Very chewy foods**: pizza crust, beef jerky, gummy bears. Note: no chewing on pencils or pens.

4. **Super sugary foods and drinks**: soda pop with sugar, ice cream, most cookies, and cake. Yes, this is the worst of the forbidden foods. Some kids will give you a tough time. But there are sugar-free versions of all these kinds of foods, to be made, baked, or store-bought.

*We* will speak about this with your son or daughter and give them a printed list, but *you* will have to reinforce, monitor, and provide some substitute foods to prevent mutiny or months of sulking. Most kids get it, though. When they understand how short or long the number of weeks of wearing braces will turn out to be, how comfortable or uncomfortable wearing them is, how maintaining hygiene while wearing them is, and how their results are linked to them staying away from the short list of harmful foods, they are pretty responsible about it. Most parents who are initially really worried about this tell us later it wasn't the horror show they'd imagined.

# Emergencies, Injuries, Travel, and Time Away from Home

Many "emergencies" actually aren't and can be easily and safely remedied at home. You are provided a guide on handling common orthodontic repairs, and you can always access the same information on our web site 24/7, 365 days/year.

Common emergencies include the breaking of some part of the braces, eating something particularly damaging—even a McDonalds bun full of sesame seeds might feel like an emergency, or, early, a feeling of discomfort that worries something serious might be wrong.

**If you do run up against an emergency that isn't easily managed with these instructions or if you can't wait for regular office hours, we have a special phone number to call that routes to a knowledgeable staff member directly and who will return your call within sixty minutes or less. You are never left out to dry.**

If your family or son or daughter are away from home and, say, they chomp down on a piece of toffee and break a piece of their braces, there is *always* a remedy. You are *not* going to cut your vacation short and rush to the airport! Again, often a remedy provided by our instructions can meet the urgent need until everybody gets back home.

## Sports

Speaking of injuries, the question of sports versus braces worries kids and parents alike. These days, kids are *very* active in organized and school sports, some starting one as another's season is ending. You know this; you are coordinating the schedules and working as their unpaid chauffeur.

Good news: for every sport and every level of play, there is either an inexpensive off-the-shelf mouth guard or a slightly costlier, custom-fit mouth guard to provide an extra, suitable level of dental protection and to protect the braces themselves. In some sports, additional face masks or other equipment normally treated as an option can be added and used during the time period of the orthodontic treatment. Ask us for guidance for your child and their sport(s). Some mouth guards even come with insurance against dental injury, covering financial costs.

We have thought this through! For example, research reported in *Clinics in Sports Medicine*—from the Department of Neurology at Boston University School of Medicine—examined uses of different kinds of mouth guards and the rate of sports-related concussions. There was no significant difference in concussion risks found tied to different types of mouth guards. We can select the best one for your child, their sport, and the level of play and, if a factor, your budget with no worry about one choice instead of another affecting risk of concussion.

This, by the way, is typical of a good orthodontic specialist: attention to *every* detail. They should have a good knowledge of every ramification of wearing braces, clinical and technological advancements, and every patient or parent need. To be blunt, it's a practical impossibility for a general dentist to give the braces work he does on the side anywhere near this same level of all-in focus.

By the way, there are collegiate and pro athletes—even NFL players—getting orthodontic treatment and even wearing braces. If they can, your child can! You do *not* need the drama of stopping your child from playing the sports they're committed to because of their orthodontic treatment.

See, this *isn't* going to be difficult!

## *Tips for Helping Your Child Adjust to a Life with Braces*

- **All the cool kids are doing it (or soon will be):** Braces are a very popular appliance during the middle school and high school years. Rather than focus on how he or she feels wearing braces, encourage your child to begin actively looking for other kids who are wearing braces. Chances are, they'll find lots more than they ever imagined!

- **Even famous people do it:** Gwen Stefani. Prince Harry. Drew Barrymore. Tom Cruise. Dakota Fanning. Danny Glover. The list of famous people who've worn braces—many of them as adults—could fill half this book. Share with your child how even the most famous people in the spotlight sometimes need a little help through braces.

- **Fast forward:** Many orthodontists provide a "before and after" consultant's session, much like a plastic surgeon. Digital pictures are often used to portray what the child's teeth might look like once the braces have been removed. Have your child focus on the "after" when he or she gets down about the "before" shots!

- **Be prepared:** Finally, create a "master list" of things your child likes to do, things that make them feel special, confident, brave, calm, relaxed, or excited. If you notice them feeling down, consult your list and make plans to do something special in the near future to boost their confidence level back to where you know it belongs!

Call us at **919-373-3656** or go to **Wilson-Ortho.com** to schedule your own Customized Smile Analysis.

# Chapter Eleven

# Life After Braces: Retainers

**SO, YOUR CHILD'S BRACES** are off and they're ready to live a life full of confidence and good oral health. They may think, *I'm free! I'm free!* Well, not quite yet.

The selection of the right braces, the expert orthodontist, and the compliant wearing of the braces gets us about three-fourths of the way to where we want to be: a well-aligned, as-perfect-as-possible, healthy smile for life.

But after braces, there are retainers.

While many patients are understandably eager to be done with braces once they come off, the fact is, retainers do as much work—if not more—than the braces themselves. Straight teeth in proper alignment have to stay that way, and for that, retainers are a big help.

When the braces are removed, teeth can still shift if not helped through a period of adjustment to settle in. Retainers gently but purposefully remind the teeth to stay straight during this adjustment period. It's advised that nearly all patients who've gone through the time, work, and expense of braces will want to use fixed or removable retainers for months or years or even for life and continue to schedule regular orthodontic checkups. Some dentists doing braces won't tell you this, but I will. Years ago, clinicians believed that once teeth were straightened by braces, they would simply stay that way forever. New science says otherwise. In fact, teeth position shifting as we age is to be expected. Teeth naturally shift to the middle and crowd. So, retainers are actually extremely important in maintaining the new smile from braces. Any claims otherwise, by some "brand" of braces or any doctor, are flat-out false.

Retainers can play a role in:

- closing any gaps that may remain in the bite

- correcting any speech problems—sometimes occurring with a new bite or jaw position

- tongue thrust—where the tongue slips under the teeth while talking

- bruxism—grinding teeth while sleeping

As you can see, there's a lot more to this than just "installing and removing braces."

In post-braces monitoring and checkups, I tend to decide on the best kind of retainer for your child before the removal of the braces. Growth of the jaw following treatment (yes, the jaw is still growing in adolescents, to age eighteen or so), stabilization of the gums and bone tissues, pressures from lips and tongue, and other factors tell me what type of retainer should be worn and for how long. Retainers are made out of rubber, plastic, and sometimes, still, metal. They are custom made and fit as part of the complete orthodontic treatment. However, after the initial orthodontic exam, at the same time the best braces are being selected, it's usually possible, with a good degree of certainty, to predict the type of retainer(s) your child is going to need, and I'm happy to share that information with you at that time.

Some retainers are invisible or nearly invisible. There are clear plastic retainers. A *fixed* retainer is typically placed on the inside/back surfaces of the lower front teeth. When your child hears "retainer" he will most likely picture a *removable* retainer. These make hygiene easy, are easily removed and cleaned daily, and can be removed for a sports activity. We will give you instructions for retainer care and maintenance. Two popular retainer cleaners are "Retainer Brite" and "Kleenite", both of which can be purchased on Amazon. In some instances, a Hawley retainer which has acrylic and a labial bow wire may be used. In my practice, we have a saying for retainer wear: "Night-time for a lifetime." Unfortunately there is no magic date we can tell patients they no longer have to wear a retainer. If retainers are not worn as prescribed, teeth will shift! It is important to know that this happens regardless of a person having their wisdom teeth or not. I can't tell you how many times I have heard that wisdom teeth caused teeth to shift, but this has not proved to be the case.

This is an important part of braces aftercare and part of the complete orthodontic treatment program personalized for your child.

Call us at **919-373-3656** or go to **Wilson-Ortho.com** to schedule your own Customized Smile Analysis.

# Chapter Twelve

# Let's Celebrate!

**HAVING TO WEAR BRACES** can last for six months to two years or more in certain cases. During the time your child has them, they may have moved from child to preteen or preteen to teen, at times feeling embarrassed by having them, and possibly missing out on some things. They probably gave up favorite foods and snacks. They at least had to be super-conscious of what they ate and didn't eat. It's been a long time since they could sink their teeth into an apple!

You endured whatever complaining there was. You traded time to the office visits. You dealt with the "uh-oh!" and the "now what did you do?" emergencies if there were any. And, of course, you paid the bill.

We like to see our patients celebrate getting their braces off. There are so many ways your child can celebrate, everything from writing a journal about their experience to recording a video that shares their experience and shows their new look.

Here are a few options your child may want to consider:

- **Throw a party**. Throwing a "braces are off" party is a great way to celebrate. They can invite their friends over, put out the foods that they've been longing for, and they can enjoy showing off those new straight teeth. Their friends will love being able to take part in the celebration.

- **Plan a photo shoot**. Your child deserves to show the world their new beautiful smile! Plan a photo shoot, so they can be one-on-one with a photographer and put their best smile forward. They'll get some great shots and can show all their friends on social media their new look.

- **Chew some gum**. Your child might have wanted to have gum for the longest time. Although it's not the best habit, they can take an afternoon to chew some gum and feel guilt and worry free. Chew to your heart's content!

- **Go caramel**. Now is the time your child can sink their teeth into something like a caramel apple. No more avoiding the caramel and cutting the apple into bite-sized pieces. Nope, they can actually eat a full caramel apple, right off the stick! They can get one at the mall or a carnival or even make one themselves. Either way, they'll love being able to bite into that sticky gooey sweetness worry free!

- **Picnic in the park**. Weather permitting, a picnic in the park will make for a fun celebration. Take some of your child's favorite outdoor games, invite the friends, and have a cooler filled with icy drinks. On the grill, you can plan for things like corn on the cob that your child had to largely avoid while wearing their braces. It will make for a memorable afternoon!

- **Have a potluck dinner**. Have your child's friends and family each bring a dish people with braces have to take precaution with. This will give them the chance to learn a little more about what you went through, and it'll be fun to see what options they come up with. Ask each of the guests to write down a comment about your child with or without her braces. Your potluck will be filled with interesting dishes, laughs, and a good time!

- **Relax**. What could be better than spending a couple of hours being pampered, or perhaps a round of golf or fishing out on the lake? Not much! Take your child out—celebrate them making it through their treatment. They'll walk out feeling and looking great!

Doing some of these things, such as chewing gum, may still not be good for your child's teeth or their body overall. But doing it on a special occasion, and not making a habit out of it, won't cause any harm.

Of course, nobody can celebrate unless we *started*. There really is no time like the present.

Call us at **919-373-3656** or go to **Wilson-Ortho.com** to schedule your own Customized Smile Analysis.

# Chapter Thirteen

# Adults and Orthodontics: How Technology Is Changing Treatment for the Better

**WHY ARE YOU PUTTING OFF** getting the smile you wish you had? Sometimes it's embarrassment; an adult considering orthodontic treatment will often say to me, "But isn't it a waste of money at this point in my life?" or "Won't people think I'm vain if I get braces now?" I guess that depends on how you'd define "waste" or "vain"—but in my experience, something as simple as getting your smile fixed can have a tremendous impact on your life, far beyond how your teeth look. Sometimes, getting that one thing fixed creates a cascade that flows into how you view yourself and your health. For example, one of my recent patients felt that cascading improvement, and in a letter to me, she wrote:

"My dentist suggested that I let Dr. Wilson see what he could do for me because I was grinding during sleep and wearing down my bottom teeth. Dr. Wilson told me about the Invisalign method.

I decided to go for it. It was the right solution for me at my age of fifty-six at the time and for my busy lifestyle.

"Soon after I started Invisalign, I started making other decisions about my health that I had not anticipated. I started dieting and walking, and soon lost fifteen pounds. I hired a concierge doctor and had a very thorough physical.

"Then, I stepped up my exercise to include running. In my three months, I lowered my cholesterol by 75 points. I hired a personal trainer who I still work with two to three times per week for ten months, and I have no plans to stop. I ran a 5K three months later. Four months later, I added cycling to my weekly routine, and I now go on rides as long seventy-five miles per day with my husband.

"Our marriage of thirty-four years is rejuvenated and my life is so great. I just celebrated my fifty-seventh birthday, and I haven't felt this good in my whole life. Thank you for Dr. Wilson and staff for kickstarting my transformation."

I don't see anything wasteful or vain in that; once you decide that you're worth it, getting that smile you've always wanted can change your whole worldview, and impact you in ways you couldn't have imagined. And it's easier than it's ever been, thanks to technology.

## What Orthodontics Used to Be, and What it is Today

If what you know about the process of moving teeth is based on your memory of how things were done when you were a kid, you'll be glad to hear that advances in science have changed everything, and very much for the better. Today's orthodontic treatments are faster, much more comfortable, and require fewer visits to the office than they used to; and progress continues at a dazzling pace.

Back when I was fourteen and needed my teeth straightened, there weren't many options available. I had standard braces. Luckily for me, I didn't require the bands on the teeth that would have called for spacers, which were quite uncomfortable. Still, these were full-on braces—the dreaded metal mouth—that used rigid steel wires to move the teeth. Even when I started practicing in the 2000s, we were still putting bands on teeth—little metal rings that went around the entire tooth—and to get them on, we had to wedge a separator or a spacer between the teeth, which without a doubt was the most painful part of orthodontics for most patients.

But nowadays, we can just glue the brace right to the tooth because the materials for bonding are so improved, so we very rarely use bands. Steel wire is largely a thing of the past too.

Office visits are far less frequent, thanks to the many new technologies we're using. When I began in practice, the doctor who I worked with had an enormous staff to service the patients coming in for their monthly visits. Today's patient can often be seen as infrequently as every eight to ten weeks.

As we discussed in chapter nine, there have been many advances to make treatment easier for patients of all ages—and thanks to their advertising, many adults come to me looking for treatment with Invisalign, and aren't always aware of the other terrific technology we've got to work with today.

For instance, taking impressions of the teeth for Invisalign was such a hassle and quite tedious. Now we can make a virtual impression using another new scanner called an iTero. This lets us get a highly accurate "impression" without goop, and in less than ten minutes. It's much easier on the patient, and we can use it as the model to fabricate Invisalign and many other orthodontic appliances. The appliances fit better and are more comfortable, too, thanks to that increased accuracy and detail.

Since many adults are concerned with their time spent in treatment, the following technologies in this chapter have the potential to reduce the overall time needed to achieve optimal results.

## Speeding Up Treatment With Technology

Another area in which treatment has been improved by technology is through devices that encourage faster tooth movement. Among the most popular are AcceleDent and the VPro5. Both work in a similar way: they apply a very light, vibrating force to the teeth. This stimulates the cells responsible for moving teeth, allowing them to work a little bit faster, and overall, minimize treatment duration. Additionally, it can also reduce the discomfort people would normally have with braces or Invisalign. When we've got a patient in our practice that needs results in a hurry—for example, someone who says, "Hey, I'm getting married next summer, can you fix my teeth?" or a college student who's graduating and needs to get their braces off by the time they're done with school—we always offer these treatments as an option to speed up their results. Recently, I had an adult patient here doing braces: we got her through treatment in just thirteen months, and she reported no pain or discomfort during the treatment. That wouldn't have been possible before.

Another newer, somewhat similar option is a machine called OrthoPulse, which works using what's called *photobiomodulation.*

This hastens treatment by delivering LED light pulses to the area around the teeth and gums to increase the blood flow, rather than using vibration as the other two do. Again, the LED light affects the cells and the bone involved in tooth movement. While it does not reduce discomfort, it does speed up results.

## What's Ahead in Orthodontics?

The biggest news in orthodontics continues to come from the advances in technology and treatment made with clear plastic aligners and 3-D printing. The technology of using plastic aligners to move teeth has been covered pretty thoroughly in this book. Suffice it to say that it's tremendously popular, especially with my adult patients, and is constantly improving in terms of what it can provide. I take a lot of continuing education courses around this technology, because there's no other way to keep up with their constant innovations.

I'm proud that Invisalign has awarded me the coveted Elite provider status, and would strongly suggest that when you're looking for a practitioner with the idea of getting Invisalign, that you choose someone who's earned that title by virtue of how many patients they have treated with the system. As in any other endeavor, practice makes perfect, and there's no good reason to trust your smile to a "weekend" practitioner. There are many practitioners who gave up on Invisalign early on, perhaps due to poor treatment results, and wrote the system itself off as flawed. Others just don't want to dedicate the time and effort necessary to become expert at it—and certainly that does require a lot of effort. But it's very clear that aligners are going to have an ever-greater part in how we move teeth in the future, and Invisalign is certainly the foremost player in this space.

# "Do It Yourself" Orthodontics? Please Don't!

One of the trends I see on the horizon is do-it-yourself (DIY) orthodontics. As counter-intuitive as it may sound, there are actually companies that are beginning to encourage consumers to cut out the practitioner altogether, and use scanning and tele-medicine to fit and order aligners from home. There are several enterprises currently pitching this idea, and while I can see why the idea of DIY orthodontics is attractive to a busy person—or to someone looking to save a little money—there's much about this notion that seems dubious to me.

For one thing, there's a lot more to moving teeth properly than simply moving them into line; if it's done wrong, you can create many more problems than you solve in terms of your bite, for instance. While I like do-it-yourself projects as much as the next person, I'd hesitate to do my own surgery because that's well outside the realm of my expertise, and because the risks so outweigh the relatively minor savings. There's a reason that orthodontists are among the most highly educated specialists out there, and why getting into an orthodontic residency is tougher, statistically, than getting into Harvard for undergraduate studies. Trust me, this is not an area in which a prudent person offers himself up as a guinea pig—and the system for self-treatment is still very much in the early stages. Added to that is the fact that retreatment for botched work can take longer and be more onerous than simply getting it done right the first time.

Your mouth matters—not just to your appearance, but also to your overall health. So much of your well-being is tied to keeping your teeth healthy and functional throughout your life. They're not an area in which you should be cutting corners. By all means, hang your own wallpaper or repair your own lawnmower—but think twice before acting as your own practitioner.

Call us at **919-373-3656** or go to **Wilson-Ortho.com** to schedule your own Customized Smile Analysis.

*"I have officially had my braces removed and I'm so pleased with how my teeth look. Dr. Wilson did a fantastic job and I will always tell anyone I know looking to straighten their teeth to go see him. Thank you so much for making life easy with the appointments and honestly just caring and understanding how important straight teeth were to me. I will forever be grateful for all you did."*

**—STEPHANIE A.**

# FAQ

Here is a handy resource guide of frequently asked questions and orthodontic terminology, many of which are answered throughout the book.

## What might happen if your child's mouth doesn't quite "fit"?

The fact is, the sooner you straighten your child's smile, the faster it will develop as it should: straight, clean, and healthy!

## Are there any celebrities who've worn braces?

Many! Gwen Stefani, Prince Harry, Drew Barrymore, Tom Cruise, Dakota Fanning, Danny Glover, and more.

## Can I see what my child's straight teeth might look like before the procedure is done?

Yes! Digital pictures are often used to portray what the child's teeth might look like once the braces have been removed.

## Will I be able to afford my child's braces?

Not only are most orthodontic procedures cheaper than ever, but insurance, payment plans, and a variety of other financing options make braces more affordable than they've ever been.

## Will getting braces be painful for my child?

Not anymore! Modern technology—and choosing the right orthodontist—can ensure that your child enjoys a pain-free orthodontic experience.

## How much school will my child miss because of braces?

Not much, actually. After initial visits and, barring the actual procedure itself, most visits and/or adjustments are routine and can take anywhere from fifteen to forty-five minutes.

## Is it really such a big deal if my child has crooked teeth?

Unfortunately, yes. Eroding, crooked, or unaligned smiles can take time to happen, but the time to act is now. Orthodontic irregularities don't just heal on their own or "go away" if you ignore them.

## What are some of the warning signs that my child might need to go to the orthodontist?

There are many, but here are a few of the most common: early or late loss of teeth, protruding teeth, grinding or clenching of teeth, and speech difficulty.

## What kind of "side effects" are caused by crooked teeth?

Some of the more frequent ones I see include headaches, tooth-aches, mouth breathing, chipped or worn down teeth, snoring, and drooling.

## What makes an orthodontist more qualified than a dentist?

Orthodontists are *dental specialists* who have completed two to three years of additional education beyond dental school to learn the proper way to align teeth and jaws.

## Why should I choose a specialist for my child's orthodontic care?

Unique treatment requirements and otherwise difficult bite problems are common, everyday scenarios for your orthodontist. In the interest of receiving the most efficient and effective orthodontic treatment possible, choose an orthodontic specialist.

## How do I know if my doctor is an orthodontist?

Only orthodontists can belong to the American Association of Orthodontists (AAO).

## What is a treatment coordinator?

During your initial consultation(s), you will usually be assigned a patient contact person—we call this person a "treatment coordinator" in our office—with whom you will schedule appointments, confer with rescheduling, and of course, answer any and all questions you may have.

## Why are follow-up visits important?

These are wonderful opportunities to either a) ask questions you may have missed the first time, or b) get further details from your orthodontist him- or herself.

## Why is early treatment so important?

Age seven is the earliest time your orthodontist can determine future jaw and tooth alignment. That's because, at the age of seven, your child's upper and lower permanent front teeth are developing. These teeth set the stage for future jaw position and serious problems can develop if they come into the wrong position.

## Is there such a thing as a child being too old for braces?

Actually, there is. Case in point: waiting to take your child to the orthodontist until they are twelve or thirteen can be very risky.

## What if I don't believe in early orthodontics?

Well, you're entitled to your opinion, but this is like saying you don't believe in the sun. You can hide from it, pretend it's not there, or refuse to acknowledge it, but the simple fact remains. If you're not aware of the potential risks, you can get burnt.

## Will my child actually need braces at seven?

Probably not. While I inform parents their child needs an initial exam at age seven, I also mention that most children *will not need braces until eleven to thirteen years of age.*

## What is a crossbite?

When the upper and lower teeth grow at different rates, or even when the lower jaw grows disproportionately with the upper jaw, something known as a "crossbite" can occur.

## Where should I start to look for treatment if I'm concerned about my child's jaw development?

If you suspect your child might have a crossbite or other issues, approach your family dentist and ask about orthodontics.

## Why should I address a crossbite?

Crossbites can lead to pain, discomfort, and lack of confidence as your child begins to feel insecure or even ostracized because of this very treatable, very normal series of jaw and teeth developments.

## What is Invisalign?

The Invisalign system is the virtually invisible way to straighten your teeth and achieve the dazzling smile you've always dreamed of. Using advanced 3-D computer-imaging technology, Invisalign depicts your complete treatment plan, from the initial position of your teeth to the final desired position.

## What are the primary benefits of Invisalign?

Like the word that inspired them, Invisalign aligners are practically clear and as close to "invisible" as one can get. No one may even notice you're wearing these virtually invisible braces, making Invisalign a seamless fit with your lifestyle and day-to-day interactions with others.

## How do I get started with Invisalign?

It's simple: just make an appointment with your local orthodontist for an initial consultation. Most doctors will offer a free initial consultation to see if you are a good candidate for Invisalign.

## How will Invisalign effectively move my teeth?

Aligners are the foundation for, and work in unison with, the Invisalign system. Like brackets and arch wires are to braces, Invisalign aligners move teeth by using the appropriate placement of controlled force on your child's teeth.

## How many patients are being treated with Invisalign?

More than five million patients worldwide have been treated with Invisalign. The number of Invisalign smiles grows daily.

## Is Invisalign appropriate for my child?

Yes, especially because Invisalign now has a system designed specifically for teens!

## How does Invisalign Teen work?

Aligners snap on your teeth easily. They are comfortable and practically invisible. Invisalign Teen allows permanent teeth to grow and gently and continuously moves your teeth in small increments. Aligners are worn for about one week, then you swap them for a new pair.

## Why are metal braces still so popular?

Metal braces are very strong and can withstand most types of treatment. Today's metal braces are smaller, sleeker, and more polished than ever before.

## Are so-called "clear braces" effective?

Ceramic braces are very strong and generally do not stain. Two popular brands are Clarity, made by 3M Unitek, and Damon Clear, made by Ormco. Adults like to choose ceramic braces because they "blend in" with the teeth and are less noticeable than metal. These are the types of braces actor Tom Cruise had.

## Are clear braces appropriate for adults?

Absolutely! Adults of all ages can enjoy the same cosmetic and health benefits of properly aligned teeth with the Damon Clear system and Clarity braces.

## What are some of my payment options in addition to insurance?

One way many patients pay for their procedures is by utilizing the benefits of what is known as "flex spending," where their employer matches their spending commitment.

## What if my child has a "braces emergency" before or after office hours?

If you are experiencing an orthodontic emergency that can't wait for regular office hours, most orthodontic offices have a special number to call, either before, during, or after business hours. If this information isn't given to you readily, ask how your doctor's office handles emergencies.

## Can a salt water rinse help deal with irritation caused by braces?

Absolutely; warm saltwater rinses soothe the cheek lining, which can get aggravated by your child's braces.

## How do I make a salt water rinse?

To make a salt water rinse, mix half a teaspoon of table salt in one cup of warm water. Stir until the salt is completely dissolved. Gently swish about a fourth of the cup in your mouth for thirty seconds. Make sure you force the water over the areas that feel sore. Then spit the water into the sink. Repeat until the entire cup is gone.

## What if my child plays sports and needs a mouth guard?

The best advice for patients or parents looking for a mouth guard can be obtained from your pediatrician, dentist, pediatric dentist, orthodontist or oral surgeon. All of these specialists are uniquely trained to offer customized advice in order to help you prevent a sports-related dental or facial injury.

## What about brushing with braces?

Here are some simple tips you can share with your child for the best results when brushing with braces on:

- Brush your teeth with a soft nylon toothbrush after you eat and before bed.

- Brush, rinse, and look; if you find any areas that are not clean, brush them again.

- Brush your gums as you brush your teeth (massage and stimulate).

- If no toothpaste is available, brush without.

- If you are unable to brush, rinse your mouth vigorously with water.

- Replace your old toothbrush when it gets worn out.

- It is absolutely essential that you continue regular visits to your family dentist for checkups and cleanings throughout your orthodontic treatment!

## What type of foods should my child avoid while wearing braces?

There are four main types of food your child should avoid while wearing braces: (1) **hard foods**, like ice, popcorn, peanut brittle, rock candy, and corn on the cob, (2) **sticky foods**, like caramels, bubble gum, taffy, and suckers, (3) **chewy foods**, like pizza crust, crusty breads, beef jerky, and gummy bears, and (4) **sugary foods and drinks**, like cake, ice cream, cookies, pie, candy, and soda pop.

## Why are retainers so important?

As we age, teeth naturally shift to the middle and crowd. Combined with late growth of the lower jaw, shifting of the teeth is expected following orthodontic treatment. Therefore, retainers are extremely important in the maintenance of your new smile following orthodontic treatment.

# Resources

Before or after your consultation, you may want more information for yourself or your son or daughter. The following websites provide valuable insight to help you make the right decision for your child.

**Braces.org** is the "all about braces site" of the American Association of Orthodontists. This is the official regulatory body and professional association of orthodontists, and *only* orthodontists (*not* dentists) can be members. Here you will receive accurate, up-to-date information on orthodontics.

**ExcellenceInOrthodontics.org** is the elite association of orthodontists subscribing to a pledge of clinical and customer services excellence. A complete collection of information for patients and parents can be found here.

# THE
# NEXT
# STEP

# Your Customized Smile Analysis

When you are ready, I urge you to schedule your Customized Smile Analysis, complete with a complimentary consultation, safe, digital x-rays (a $249 value) an exam, and a report provided to you and your son or daughter—all without cost or obligation.

Call us at **919-373-3656** or go to **Wilson-Ortho.com**.